PHARMACY RX TRAINER
STUDENT WORKBOOK

Christie E. Martin, MSM, CPhT

Federico Lopez, CPhT

Sterile Solutions, VP

JONES AND BARTLETT PUBLISHERS

Sudbury, Massachusetts

BOSTON   TORONTO   LONDON   SINGAPORE

World Headquarters

Jones and Bartlett Publishers
40 Tall Pine Drive
Sudbury, MA 01776
978-443-5000
info@jbpub.com
www.jbpub.com

Jones and Bartlett Publishers
Canada
6339 Ormindale Way
Mississauga, Ontario L5V 1J2
Canada

Jones and Bartlett Publishers
International
Barb House, Barb Mews
London W6 7PA
United Kingdom

Jones and Bartlett's books and products are available through most bookstores and online booksellers. To contact Jones and Bartlett Publishers directly, call 800-832-0034, fax 978-443-8000, or visit our website www.jbpub.com.

Substantial discounts on bulk quantities of Jones and Bartlett's publications are available to corporations, professional associations, and other qualified organizations. For details and specific discount information, contact the special sales department at Jones and Bartlett via the above contact information or send an email to specialsales@jbpub.com.

The authors, editor, and publisher have made every effort to provide accurate information. However, they are not responsible for errors, omissions, or for any outcomes related to the use of the contents of this book and take no responsibility for the use of the products and procedures described. Treatments and side effects described in this book may not be applicable to all people; likewise, some people may require a dose or experience a side effect that is not described herein. Drugs and medical devices are discussed that may have limited availability controlled by the Food and Drug Administration (FDA) for use only in a research study or clinical trial. Research, clinical practice, and government regulations often change the accepted standard in this field. When consideration is being given to use of any drug in the clinical setting, the health care provider or reader is responsible for determining FDA status of the drug, reading the package insert, and reviewing prescribing information for the most up-to-date recommendations on dose, precautions, and contraindications, and determining the appropriate usage for the product. This is especially important in the case of drugs that are new or seldom used.

Production Credits
Publisher: David Cella
Editorial Assistant: Maro Asadoorian
Production Manager: Julie Champagne Bolduc
Production Assistant: Jessica Steele Newfell
Associate Marketing Manager: Lisa Gordon
Manufacturing and Inventory Control Supervisor: Amy Bacus
Composition: Shawn Girsberger
Cover Design: Kate Ternullo
Cover Image: © Rob Byron/ShutterStock, Inc.
Printing and Binding: Courier Stoughton
Cover Printing: Courier Stoughton

ISBN 978-0-7637-6914-7

6048

Printed in the United States of America
16 15 14 13 12   10 9 8 7 6 5 4 3

This book is dedicated to our families for their unwavering support.

This book is dedicated to our students, whom we love dearly.

This book is dedicated to our partnership and our friendship, which we will cherish forever.

CONTENTS

Preface. vii

SECTION I   **Introduction to Pharmacy Lab**. 1
Sig Codes and Abbreviations. 1
Translating Sig Code Worksheet 4
Pharmacy Conversions 5
Conversions Activity 7
Controlled Substances 8
Identifying Controlled Substances 10
Drug References 12
Drug References Riddle Worksheet 14

SECTION II   **Working Retail Pharmacy** **15**
Data Entry 15
Sample Patient Profile 17
Receiving the Prescription 18
Parts of the Prescription 19
Parts of the Sig Code 20
What Is Missing Activity Worksheet 22
Day's Supply 27
DEA Verification 30
Determining Valid DEA Numbers 32
DEA Verification Activity 36
Writing Prescriptions 37
Assembly 38
8-Point Check Activity 42
Exceptions 46
Completing a Refill Request Form 49
Insurance Card Activity 53
Insurance Rejections 53
Telephone Etiquette 56
Telephone Etiquette Activity 58

SECTION III   **Working Hospital Pharmacy** **59**

Medication Administration Record 59

Formulary 61

Formulary Activity 61

Unit Dosing 62

Unit-Dose–Filling Activity 62

Intravenous Lab 63

Hand Washing 63

Horizontal and Vertical Laminar Flow Hoods 64

Needles and Syringes 65

Preparation of Chemotherapy IVs 68

Small- and Large-Volume Parenterals 69

Labeling Intravenous Drugs 70

Batching and Pre-Packing 71

SECTION IV   **Special Topics in Pharmacy** **73**

Ethics in Pharmacy: A Class Discussion 73

Pharmacy Technician Law: A Quick Guide 75

Pharmacy Law Activity 77

Medication Errors 78

Medication Errors Online Activity 78

HIV: How Much Do You Know? 79

Sexual Harassment on the Job 81

Discrimination at Work 82

Prescription Samples **83**

The Converter Tool **101**

PREFACE

Chances are—if you are reading this book—you are looking for something to help you train better and smarter as a pharmacy technician. If you are a teacher, this workbook can help you structure your laboratory setting. If you are a student, you will reap the benefits of the activities found in this workbook. The application of what you learn here will help you when you finally begin working as a pharmacy technician.

This workbook is accompanied by software that will aid instructors teaching pharmacy technician students in an educational setting and will allow students to get the feel for what inputting prescriptions is really like. To order this software, please visit http://www.jbpub.com/catalog/9780763760328.

Our vision was to design affordable software that pharmacy technician program educators could use to enhance the student learning experience. It is training software made simple.

- Being Internet-based makes it available to virtually anyone with an Internet connection. There are no expensive monthly fees associated with its purchase.
- Screens are easy to follow, even if you have no experience.
- The program is user-friendly and very straightforward.

As educators, we have found that students learn best when all five senses are engaged. This software provides real-world hands-on manipulation that enables students to:

- Input prescriptions
- Practice using common abbreviations
- Enhance brand and generic name recognition
- Develop patient profile utilization
- Print a prescription label

Students will have the opportunity to practice:

- Receiving the prescription
- Typing the prescription
- Filling the prescription
- Labeling prescription bottles

These are all components found in a real pharmacy. Instructors can now run laboratory sessions like an actual pharmacy. Students will feel confident going out into the field fully prepared. The intent of this software is to encourage and develop foundational pharmacy skills. Developing and practicing these skills will aid in meeting the needs of the ever-changing world of pharmacy. The software can be used individually, or in a small network group of computers. We recommend spending time on it individually as well as in group settings. Many of the activities are intended for collaborative learning situations.

The pharmacy training software is a realistic computer database that the student can use to practice entering patient information and patient prescriptions. There are drugs and commonly used pharmacy codes pre-entered into the software. Instructors and students have the option of inputting any new drugs or codes for their own purposes. The software includes outpatient, inpatient, and unit dose labeling capabilities. Also included are doctor and insurance information tabs. The software prints labels from virtually any printer. Label paper can be purchased through www.pharmex.com or by calling 1-800-233-0585. Using the FlickAway PXT-5M version will print the sample labels found in this workbook. We welcome suggestions from instructors and students alike to upgrade software and modify activities in order to enhance learning. Instructor resources will be provided online.

Thank you for giving us the opportunity to enhance your training.

Acknowledgments

We would like to thank Jones and Bartlett Publishers for facilitating the production of this workbook. Mike Brown, Dave Cella, and Royal Hale provided their expertise and shared valuable insights in the development phase. This experience has empowered us to make a difference in the lives of students as well as in our own. Thank you to all.

INTRODUCTION TO PHARMACY LAB

I

Sig Codes and Abbreviations

Pharmacy technicians must be able to read prescriptions and doctor's orders. In order to do that, pharmacy technicians must learn to understand words and codes that are rooted in Greek and Latin. As a pharmacy technician, you will be learning *sig codes* to translate the doctor's orders and prescriptions patients bring to your pharmacy. Learning the meaning of these abbreviations will enable the pharmacy technician to enter data quickly and accurately. The data entry technician who receives the prescription sets the pace for the entire pharmacy. This is a very important task, and employers prefer to hire technicians who know the sig codes and who can work quickly and efficiently. Using the flashcards at the back of the lab workbook will help you study and remember these common sig codes used in a pharmacy.

Use the training software to practice reading and inputting sig codes from the prescriptions in the back of this workbook. This will not only help you learn and memorize your sig codes but will help you learn the dispensing process required to fill prescriptions on the job. Remember that you must create a patient profile for each new patient. Review the information in Section II on patient profiles. Your instructor may provide you with additional prescriptions to input into the system; this practice will help you learn the sig codes and abbreviations and will increase your proficiency and speed.

1

Routes

ad	right ear
as	left ear
au	both ears
im	intramuscular
iv	intravenous
ivpb	intravenous piggyback
od	right eye
os	left eye
ou	both eyes
pc	after meals (food)
po	orally (by mouth)
pr	rectally
prn	as needed
pv	vaginally
sl	sublingually
supp	suppository
top	topically

Frequency

ac	before meals
am	morning
bid	two times a day
hs	at bedtime
qam	every morning
qd	once a day
qh	every hour
qid	four times a day
qod	every other day
qpm	every evening
q 4°–6°	every 4 to 6 hours
stat	now / immediately
tid	three times a day

Measurements

cc	cubic centimeter
gm	gram
gr	grain
gtt	drop
hr	hour
L	liter
lb	pound
mcg	microgram
mEq	milliequivalent
mg	milligram
ml	milliliter
mm	millimeter
oz	ounce
ss	one half
Tbsp	tablespoon
tsp	teaspoon

Dosage Forms

cap	capsule
crm	cream
sr, xl, xr	extended release
supp	suppository
syr	syrup
tab	tablet
ung	ointment

Miscellaneous

aa	of each
apap	acetaminophen
app	applicator
asa	aspirin (acetylsalicylic acid)
bp	blood pressure
c	with
d/c	discontinue
hctz	hydrochlorothaizide
htn	hypertension
inj	inject
ms	morphine sulfate
nr	no refill
ns	normal saline
pcn	penicillin
qs	quantity sufficient or "up to"
sig	directions
tcn	tetracycline
ud	as directed
uti	urinary tract infection

TRANSLATING SIG CODE WORKSHEET

Practice translating the following sig codes. Below each sentence write down the translation as the patient would read it on his or her prescription bottle. After reviewing Section II, come back to this worksheet and decide which verb should be used for each.

1. i-ii tab po q8–12h prn muscle spasm

2. ii gtts as q4–6h prn pain

3. ii puffs po bid prn asthma sx

4. i tab po qd × 3 days then increase i tab bid

5. i tab po at onset HA MR 1 × after 2h if no relief

6. i tab po 7am, 1 tab noon, 1/2 tab 4pm

7. i tab po qid ac & hs

8. ii tab po bid-tid prn congestion

9. i supp pr q6h prn n/v

10. i applicatorful vag hs × 7 nights

Pharmacy Conversions

In addition to sig codes and abbreviations, you must also be familiar with conversions. Pharmacy uses several different measuring systems, such as the apothecary system, the household system, and the metric system. It is important for the pharmacy technician to be able to use each system accurately and convert between systems. The following charts will give you an overview of the common conversions you will need to begin working in a pharmacy.

Weight		*Volume*	
1 kg	1000 gm	1 L	1000 ml
1 gm	1000 mg	1 pt	473 ml
1 mg	1000 mvg	1 qt	946 ml
1 lb	454 gm	1 ml	1 cc
1 kg	2.2 lbs	1 gal	3785 ml
1 oz	30 gm (dry)	1 m	15 gtt
1 gr	60 mg or 65 mg	1 pt	16 oz
1 lb	16 oz	1 qt	32 oz
		1 fl oz	30 ml (liquid)
		1 gal	4 qt
		1 pt	473 ml
		1 qt	2 pt
		1 tsp	5 ml
		1 Tbsp	15 ml

Temperature Conversions

A pharmacy technician must know how to convert between the two scales used for temperature, degrees Celsius and degrees Fahrenheit, abbreviated as °C and °F. The Celsius scale is based on the freezing and boiling points of water; the freezing point is 0°C, and the boiling point is 100°C. On the Fahrenheit scale, the freezing point of water is 32°F and the boiling point is 212°F.

The formula to convert between Celsius and Fahrenheit is:

$$°C = \frac{5°F - 160}{9}$$

Celsius to Fahrenheit

To convert 80°F to Celsius, replace the "F" with 80:

$$°C = \frac{5(80) - 160}{9}$$

Remember to multiply a number inside of parentheses by the number outside of the parentheses; in this case, multiply 5 by 80.

$$°C = \frac{400 - 160}{9}$$

Next, subtract 160 from 400.

$$°C = \frac{240}{9}$$

Finally, divide 240 by 9. The answer is °C = 26.7

Fahrenheit to Celsius

To convert 30°C to Fahrenheit, replace the C with 30:

$$30 = \frac{5°F - 160}{9}$$

Multiply both sides by 9:

$$9 \times 30 = 5°F - 160$$

Add 160 to both sides:

$$270 + 160 = 5°F - 160 + 160$$

Divide both sides by 5:

$$\frac{430}{5} = \frac{5°F}{5}$$

The answer is 86 = F

Use the conversion tool in the back of this workbook to help you learn conversions. Use the tool by sliding the inner tab to what you desire to convert. For example, if you slide the inner tab to 1 gm in the first box, the second box will show 1000 mg.

CONVERSIONS ACTIVITY

Figure out the correct conversion for each of the following. Remember that you may have to convert twice to get to the right answer.

1. 3 kg = _____lb

2. 946 ml = _____pt

3. 2 gal = _____ml

4. 3 gr = _____mg

5. 60 gtts = _____ml

6. 0.008 L = _____ml

7. 20ml = _____tsp

8. 66 lb = _____kg

9. 2 Tbsp = _____ml

10. 240 ml = _____oz

Controlled Substances

The Controlled Substances Act of 1970 (CSA) classifies drugs according to their medical usefulness and their potential for addiction or harm. The CSA resulted in the creation of the Drug Enforcement Administration (DEA). There are five classes of drugs. The DEA has determined that Class I substances, also known as Schedule I substances, have no accepted medical use and/or the greatest potential for abuse or addiction. It is important to recognize a prescription for a controlled substance, because there can be many legal issues. It is the responsibility of the pharmacy technician to be aware of the laws governing the state in which he or she works. The following is an abbreviated list of controlled substances by schedule; the complete lists are available at the DEA Web site (www.usdoj.gov/dea).

Schedule I

Highest abuse potential. No accepted medicinal uses in the United States.

- Marijuana
- Lysergic acid diethylamide (LSD)
- GHB gamma (hydroxybutyric acid)

Schedule II

Less abuse potential than Schedule I. Some medicinal uses. High potential for abuse or addiction. Must be written on a special prescription pad. Prescription must be filled within 7 days. No refills permitted.

- Adderall (amphetamine and dextroamphetamine)
- Ritalin (methylphenidate)
- Concerta (methylphenidate)
- Oxycontin (oxycodone)
- Demerol (meperidine)
- Duragesic (fentanyl)

Schedule III

Less abuse potential than Schedule II. Substantial risk of abuse or addiction. Must be filled within 6 months of the written date. Can be refilled 5 times.

- Vicodin (hydrocodone and acetaminophen)
- Lortab (hydrocodone and acetaminophen)
- Norco (hydrocondone and acetaminophen)
- Vicodin ES (hydrocodone and acetaminophen)

Schedule IV

Less abuse potential than Schedule III. May be habit-forming or addictive. Must be filled within 6 months of the written date. Can be refilled 5 times.

- Valium (diazepam)

- Ativan (lorazepam)

- Klonopin (clonazepam)

- Xanax (alprazolam)

- Dalmane (flurazepam)

- Restoril (temazepam)

- Serax (oxazepam)

- Versed (midazolam)

Schedule V

Less abuse potential than Schedule IV. May be addictive or habit-forming. Must be filled within 6 months of the written date. Prescription can be refilled 5 times. May be purchased without a prescription in some states.

- Robitussin AC (guaifenesin and codeine)

- Lomotil (diphenoxylate and atropine)

- Kapectolin PG (bismuth subsalicy)

- Motofen (difenoxin and atropine)

Individual States

Individual states may add drugs to the list of controlled substances at the discretion of their state boards of pharmacy. For example, the DEA does not list Soma (carisoprodol), a skeletal muscle relaxant, as a controlled substance by the DEA, but several states—including Alabama, Arizona, Arkansas, Florida, Georgia, Hawaii, Indiana, Kentucky, Minnesota, New Mexico, Oklahoma, Oregon, and West Virginia—do consider it a controlled substance. State boards of pharmacy may move controlled substances to a higher class (for example, a drug may be reclassified from Schedule V to Schedule III), but they may not move a controlled substance to a lower class.

IDENTIFYING CONTROLLED SUBSTANCES

Use available references, such as *Drug Facts and Comparisons*, the *PDR*, or the Internet, to find a controlled substance from each of the five classes. List indications (what the drug is used for), dosage forms, side effects, and dosing information. If the drug has more than one indication, list the dosing information for only one of the indications.

Schedule I (Class I)

Drug name: _____

Indications: _____

Dosage forms: _____

Side effects: _____

Standard dosing: _____

Schedule II (Class II)

Drug name: _____

Indications: _____

Dosage forms: _____

Side effects: _____

Standard dosing: _____

Schedule III (Class III)

Drug name: _____

Indications: _____

Dosage forms: _____

Side effects: _____

Standard dosing: _____

Schedule IV (Class IV)

Drug name: _____

Indications: _____

Dosage forms: _____

Side effects: _____

Standard dosing: _____

Schedule V (Class V)

Drug name: _____

Indications: _____

Dosage forms: _____

Side effects: _____

Standard dosing: _____

Drug References

Pharmacy technicians use multiple sources for information on medications, and there are many pharmacy reference books available. In the pages that follow, you will discover a variety of reference material. Here you should take the time to understand how each reference book is used in pharmacy practice.

American Drug Index

- ✓ Facts and comparisons of drug information
- ✓ Monographs of drug products, practical equivalents, normal laboratory values, trademark glossary, container requirements, oral dosage information, and drug names that look alike

Drug Facts and Comparisons

- ✓ Provides comprehensive information about drugs available in the United States, including action, indications, contraindications, warnings, precautions, adverse reactions, administration, and dosage information

Drug Topics Red Book

- ✓ Lists more than 150,000 prescription drugs
- ✓ Over-the-counter medications
- ✓ Latest pricing information
- ✓ Trademarked names
- ✓ Generic cross-references
- ✓ NDC numbers

Martindale: The Complete Drug Reference

- ✓ Comprehensive information on drugs and medicines used throughout the world
- ✓ Includes drugs in clinical use, veterinary and investigational agents, other compounds used in medicine, herbal medicines, and toxic substances

Merck Index

- ✓ Provides concise descriptions of more than 10,000 organic and inorganic chemicals, drugs, and biological substances
- ✓ Includes formulas, alternate names, physical properties, uses, toxicity, and journal and patent references

➤ *Orange Book*

✓ Identifies drug products approved on the basis of safety and effectiveness by the Food and Drug Administration under the Federal Food, Drug, and Cosmetic Act

✓ Lists of approved generic equivalences

▲ *Physicians' Desk Reference (PDR)*

✓ Includes essential information on major pharmaceutical and diagnostic products

✓ Includes appearance, composition, action, use, dosage, and side effects

✓ 4000 drugs by product and generic name, manufacturer, and category

Remington: The Science and Practice of Pharmacy

✓ Presented in eight parts covering orientation, pharmaceutics, pharmaceutical chemistry, testing/analysis/control, pharmacokinetics and pharmacodynamics, pharmaceutical and medicinal agents, pharmaceutical manufacturing, and pharmacy practice

✓ Also used widely by pharmacists

U.S. Pharmacopeia–National Formulary

✓ Official compendium of drug information from the United States Pharmacopeial Convention

✓ Presented in official monographs of information about drug substances and dosage forms, pharmaceutical ingredients, and drug standards

USP Dictionary of Drug Names

✓ Annual list of drug nonproprietary names, brand names, chemical abstracts registry numbers, molecular and graphic formulas, and code designations

DRUG REFERENCES RIDDLE WORKSHEET

Which pharmacy reference is used in the following riddles?

Riddle Clue:
Known as the bible of pharmacy, this book will suit any technician's fancy.

_____

Riddle Clue:
This book is the color of an apple and is very pricey.

_____

Riddle Clue:
Rhymes with nightingale and holds information about drugs around the world.

_____

Riddle Clue:
The doctor may need a rest after reading this book that has 4000 drug products.

_____

Riddle Clue:
Safety is the key to this book approved by the FDA.

_____

Riddle Clue:
Special formulas and over 10,000 chemicals found in this book will have you going berserk.

_____

Riddle Clue:
Used by pharmacists, this book is divided into eight parts.

_____

Riddle Clue:
UPS delivers packages, but this book delivers a list of nationally used drugs.

_____

As an activity, get into pairs and come up with your own riddles to help you learn your drug references!

WORKING
RETAIL PHARMACY

II

Data Entry

Patient Profiles

Each new patient must fill out a patient profile. It is very important for the information to be correct. The patient will not always be the person dropping off the prescription; the patient may be a child; or the patient may be too sick to come in to the pharmacy.

The patient's name is the obvious place to start; be sure to confirm the correct spelling. Ask whether the patient has a middle initial or a suffix such as Jr., Sr., or III. The patient's date of birth is very important, because it is useful in preventing medication errors when more than one patient at the pharmacy has the same name.

The sex of the patient is also important. Some medications may be prescribed to only one sex, such as oral contraceptives, and some medications should not be handled by women who may be pregnant. Do not try to guess the sex of the patient from the patient's name. Some names are not gender specific, such as Leslie, Stacy, Sam, Tracy, or Dana, or the name may be from a culture with which you are unfamiliar, such as Thu, Van, Harwinder, or Illya.

The patient's address is necessary to fill controlled medications; some pharmacy software will not allow you to fill a controlled prescription if the address information is missing. Most patients will not have a problem providing their address. If a patient is reluctant, you can explain that federal privacy and confidentiality regulations (HIPAA) prevent the pharmacy from sharing patient information, including addresses. A phone number is necessary in order to contact the patient in case of a problem with the patient's prescription or in case of a drug recall. Any reliable contact number is acceptable, as long as the pharmacy is able to reach the patient.

It is extremely important to record and confirm drug allergies. It is good practice to ask patients about allergies every time they drop off a new prescription, as they may have developed a new allergy since the last time they received a prescription. Doctors may overlook a drug allergy or the patient may see a new doctor and forget to mention a drug allergy.

A list of the patient's medical conditions is necessary, because some medications can interact with medical conditions. For example, patients with high blood pressure should not take decongestants, because decongestants can raise blood pressure. Similarly, it is important to record all medications a patient is taking, to prevent drug interactions. Make sure to include over-the-counter drugs, prescription drugs, vitamins and supplements, and herbal remedies.

Older patients sometimes have a difficult time with childproof caps, because they may have developed arthritis or they may have lost strength and dexterity in their hands. In these cases, the patient may request EZ-Open caps, which pop off easily. Your pharmacy may require the patient to sign a waiver, depending on the laws in your state.

Keep in mind that some of your patients may not speak English. For example, cities along the border between the United States and Mexico may have patients who speak only Spanish and therefore only read Spanish. Some pharmacy software automatically translates prescription directions into Spanish if the technician indicates on the patient's profile that he or she speaks Spanish.

Use the training software and input your classmates as patients in the online pharmacy. This will give you good practice on what questions to ask and input when creating a patient profile. Use the following sample patient profile and make up the required information.

SAMPLE PATIENT PROFILE

Training Pharmacy

3001 Appletree Boulevard

San Antonio, TX 78251

Phone: 210-559-9987 Fax: 210-559-9988

PATIENT PROFILE

Last name:_____ First name: _____

Middle initial:_____ Suffix (Jr., Sr., III, etc.): _____

Date of birth (MM/DD/YYYY): _____ Sex (M/F):_____

Address:_____

City: _____ State:_____ Zip: _____

Home phone: _____ Cell: _____ Work: _____

Drug allergies: _____

_____

Medical conditions: _____

_____

_____

Other medications patient is taking (OTC, RX, Herbal): _____

_____

_____

EZ-Open (Y/N): _____ Language: _____

Receiving the Prescription

If a patient is dropping off a prescription and is new to your pharmacy, he or she will fill out a new patient profile. The form should request all of the information needed. Even if the patient has been to the pharmacy before, there is still important information that the technician will need to gather and write on the front of the prescription. *Never* write in the area where the drug and directions are written.

1. Verify the patient's name. If it is not written clearly, rewrite it.
2. The patient's date of birth should always be written on the prescription, especially if there are two patients with same name who fill prescriptions at the pharmacy.
3. Ask the patient if the generic brand is acceptable. If you are not sure whether the drug has a generic form, you may say something like, "If this drug has a generic available, is the generic brand OK?"
4. Especially if the patient is not going to be waiting in the pharmacy for the prescription, be sure to get a contact number in case a problem occurs with filling the prescription.
5. Ask each patient about drug allergies every time the patient drops off a prescription. Patients can develop new allergies, especially as they are prescribed new drugs.

Parts of the Prescription

John Smith, MD
1234 Medical Drive
San Antonio, TX 78231

❶ Phone: 210-555-1234   **Fax:** 210-555-1235

❷ Patient name: *Jane Doe*   **❸ Date:** *08/05/*

Address: *123 Drury Lane San Antonio, TX 78231*

❹ *Amoxil 875mg*

❺ *#30*

❻ *1 tab po tid x 10 days*

❼ Refills: *0*

❽ Dr.'s signature: *John Smith, MD*   **DEA #:** *AS123456*

❶ Doctor's name, office address, and phone number
❷ Patient's name and address
❸ Written date
❹ Drug name and strength
❺ Quantity to be dispensed
❻ Directions to the patient
❼ Refills
❽ Doctor's signature and DEA number (if the prescription is a controlled substance)

Parts of the Sig Code

John Smith, MD
1234 Medical Drive
San Antonio, TX 78231

Phone: 210-555-1234   **Fax:** 210-555-1235

Patient name: *Jane Doe*   **Date:** *08/05/*

Address: *123 Drury Lane San Antonio, TX 78231*

Amoxil 875mg

#30

1 tab po tid x 10 days

Refills: *0*

Dr.'s signature: *John Smith, MD*   **DEA #:** *AS123456*

In the prescription on the preceding page, the sig is written in shorthand using sig codes. *Sig* means directions to the patient. Remember that as a pharmacy technician part of your job will be to interpret sig codes and translate the directions into plain English so that the patient can understand how to take the medication. Review the sig codes in Section I. When translating a prescription, it is important to use proper grammar and punctuation and to write complete sentences. When translated, the above directions should read as follows:

Take one tablet by mouth 3 times daily for 10 days.

All directions are made up of six parts: verb, quantity, form, route, frequency, and special directions. The directions for this prescription are broken down as follows:

Take	one	tablet	by mouth	3 times daily	for 10 days
Verb	Quantity	Form	Route	Frequency	Special

- Verb: Always start directions with a verb. Verbs used with prescriptions include: take, give, apply, inject, use, instill (used for drops), place, inhale, spray, wash, swish and spit, swish and swallow, insert.

- Quantity: The amount that will be taken, given, injected, inserted, etc. Can be any number, including whole numbers (1, 5, 15), fractions (½), and decimals (3.5)

- Form: Can be the dosage form or a unit of measure, such as tablets, capsules, suppositories, ml's, or cc's.

- Route: How the medication will be taken, given, injected, inserted, etc. Examples include: by mouth, topically, nasally, right eye, left eye, right ear, left ear, vaginally, rectally.

- Frequency: How often the medication will be used. Examples include: daily, twice daily, every other day, every 4 to 6 hours, every 12 hours, after meals, at bedtime.

- Special: Used to clarify the directions further. Some examples include: as needed for pain, for 10 days, while awake, for hypertension.

WHAT IS MISSING ACTIVITY WORKSHEET

Read the following prescriptions and determine what information is missing. Use the spaces below to write down your answers.

John Smith, MD
1234 Medical Drive
San Antonio, TX 78231

Phone: 210-555-1234   **Fax:** 210-555-1235

Patient name: _Jane Doe_   **Date:** _____

Address: _123 Drury Lane San Antonio, TX 78231_

Augmentin 875mg

_#30_

1 tab po tid x 10 days

Dr.'s signature: _John Smith, MD_   **DEA #:** _AS123456_

_____

_____

_____

Joan Miller, MD

Phone: 210-532-0987   **Fax:** 210-525-9877

Patient name: _Joseph Fiennes_   **Date:** _08/05/_

Address: _209 Theater Avenue Chicago, IL 44987_

Prozac 20 mg

#30

1 tab po qhs

Refills: _1_

Dr.'s signature: _____ **DEA #:** _AS123456_

Herbert Lewis, MD
3456 Pasteur Boulevard
Los Angeles, CA 90231

Phone: 908-222-0090   **Fax:** 908-222-0098

Patient name:_____ **Date:** _08/05/_

Address: _2988 Birch Trail Los Angeles, CA 90231_____

Tylenol # 3

#30

1 tab po qd

Refills:_1_

_____

Dr.'s signature: _Herbert Lewis, MD_____ **DEA #:**_____

Robert Kelley, MD
8976 Mulberry Lane
San Antonio, TX 78231

Phone: 210-667-8975   **Fax:** 210-555-1235

Patient name: _Alicia Griffon_   **Date:** _08/05/_

Address:

Albuterol MDI

#1 unit

Refills: _3_

Dr.'s signature: _Robert Kelley, MD_   **DEA #:** _AS123456_

1234 Medical Drive
San Antonio, TX 78231

Phone: 210-555-1234   **Fax:** 210-555-1235

Patient name: _Angela_ _____ **Date:** _____

Address: _3765 Lilly Pond_ _____

Vicodin 500mg

#20

1 tab po q4-6 hours prn pain

Refills: _0_

Dr.'s signature: _____ **DEA #:** _____

Day's Supply

When translating prescriptions you will have to calculate a day supply. A day supply indicates how many days the medication will last for the patient, based on the total amount of medication given and how much medication the patient takes per day. A correct day supply is important for insurance claims and also to ensure the patient is taking the medications correctly. Some day supplies will be easier to calculate than others, but with some practice you will be able to calculate any day supply.

To calculate a day supply, divide the total number of units the patient receives by the number of units the patient takes per day. Units can be tablets, capsules, doses, ml, cc, etc.

Example 1

Drug: Lipitor 10 mg
Qty: 30 tablets
Directions: Take 1 tablet by mouth daily.
Total number of units the patient receives is 30.
The number of units the patient takes per day is 1, and 30 divided by 1 = 30 days.

Example 2

Drug: Amoxicillin 500 mg
Qty: 30 capsules
Directions: Take 1 capsule by mouth 3 times daily.
The total number of units the patient receives is 30.
The patient takes 3 units per day (1 capsule 3 times daily, $1 \times 3 = 3$), and 30 divided by 3 is 10 days.

Example 3

Drug: Vicodin 5/500 mg
Qty: 36 tablets
Directions: Take 1 to 2 tablets by mouth every 4 to 6 hours as needed for pain.
The total number of units the patient receives is 36.
The patient can take 1 to 2 tablets. Always assume the patient will take the maximum dosage; in this case, 2 tablets. The patient can take the medication every 4 to 6 hours. Always assume the patient will take the medication as often as possible; in this case, every 4 hours. If the patient takes the medication every 4 hours, he or she will take the medication 6 times in one day (24 hours divided by 4 hours = 6). The number of units the patient takes per day is 12 (2 tablets 6 times daily, $2 \times 6 = 12$), and 36 divided by 12 = 3 days.

Example 4

Drug: Flonase nasal spray
Qty: 6.7 ml (120 metered doses)
Directions: Use 2 sprays in each nostril daily.
The total number of units the patient receives is 6.7 ml, or 120 metered sprays.
Inhalers provide the amount in milliliters or grams as well as the number of doses in each inhaler. Use the number of doses in each inhaler to calculate the day supply. Also remember that patients have two nostrils as well as two eyes and two ears.
The number of units the patient takes per day is 4 (2 sprays in each nostril, which is 4 sprays daily, 4 $\times$ 1 = 4); 120 doses divided by 4 per day = 30 days.

Example 5

Drug: Tussionex suspension
Qty: 4 ounces
Directions: Take 1 teaspoonful every 12 hours.
The total number of units the patient receives is 4 ounces, which is 120 ml.
Prescriptions for liquids such as suspensions, syrups, and elixirs are usually written in ounces and the directions in teaspoons or tablespoons. Convert to ml in order to calculate the correct day supply. Using the conversion tool, convert both the ounces and teaspoon to milliliters: 4 ounces = 120 ml, and 1 teaspoon = 5 ml. The number of units the patient takes per day is 10 ml (1 teaspoon, which is 5 ml, every 12 hours, which is 2 times daily, 5 $\times$ 2 = 10), and 120 divided by 10 = 12 days.

Example 6

Drug: Cipro Otic drops
Qty: 5 ml
Directions: Instill 3 drops into right ear 4 times daily.
The total number of units the patient receives is 5ml, which is 75 drops.
Prescriptions for ear drops and eye drops are written in ml, and the directions are written in drops. Convert to milliliters in order to calculate the correct day supply. Using the conversion tool, follow the directions to convert milliliters to drops: 5 ml = 75 drops. The total number of units the patient takes per day is 12 drops (3 drops in right ear 4 times daily, 3 $\times$ 4 = 12), and 75 drops divided by 12 per day = 6.25, which, rounded to the whole number, is 6 days.
You will not be able to calculate all-day supplies; sometimes you will have to verify with the pharmacist what to use.

Example 7

Drug: Bactroban cream
Qty: 30 gm
Directions: Apply to affected area twice daily.

In this case, although the prescription provides the total number of units that the patient will receive, it does not provide the number of units that the patient will use per day. The prescription also does not describe how large the affected area is: it could be a small area, such as an ear lobe, or it could be a large area, such as the entire back. In cases like these, the pharmacy technician should ask the pharmacist to determine a day supply. Some pharmacies may have standards that technicians should follow.

DEA Verification

The Drug Enforcement Agency is charged with preventing the diversion of controlled substance for illicit purposes, in other words, preventing controlled substances from being sold to people for other than medical purposes. Doctors who want to prescribe controlled substances must apply for a DEA number; this number is part of the DEA's system to prevent diversion of controlled substances. A DEA number has the following characteristics:

1. Consists of nine alphanumeric characters, in the form of two letters followed by seven numbers.
2. The first letter will be "A" or "B."
3. The second letter will be the first letter of the prescriber's last name.
4. The seventh number is the means by which the validity of the DEA number can be checked.

Pharmacy technicians must verify DEA numbers to protect the pharmacy from fraudulent prescriptions. Examine the following prescription for a controlled substance.

John Smith, MD
1234 Medical Drive
San Antonio, TX 78231

Phone: 210-555-1234   **Fax:** 210-555-1235

Patient name: _Jane Doe_   **Date:** _08/05/_

Address: _123 Drury Lane San Antonio, TX 78231_

Vicodin 5/500mg

#30

1-2 tab po q4-6h prn pain

Refills: _0_

Dr.'s signature: _John Smith, MD_   **DEA #:** _AS1986213_

As noted, all DEA numbers will begin with an "A" or "B," followed by the first letter of the doctor's last name. In this prescription, Dr. Smith's DEA number begins with the letters "A" and "S."

To confirm the validity of the number, examine the seven digits; the numbers in Dr. Smith's DEA number are "1986213." Add the first, third, and fifth numbers.

1	9	8	6	2	1	3
1st	2nd	3rd	4th	5th	6th	7th

$$1 + 8 + 2 = 11$$

Then, add the second, fourth, and sixth numbers, and multiply the result by 2.

1	9	8	6	2	1	3
1st	2nd	3rd	4th	5th	6th	7th

$$9 + 6 + 1 = 16$$

$$16 \times 2 = 32$$

Add the answer from the first calculation to the answer from the last calculation.

$$11 + 32 = 43$$

The last digit should be the seventh digit of the doctor's DEA number, a 3 in this case. The last digit of Dr. Smith's DEA number, AS1986213, is 3, so this DEA number is valid.

DETERMINING VALID DEA NUMBERS

For the following prescriptions, write down all the pertinent information needed to begin the dispensing process. Only determine the validity of the DEA number if the prescription is for a controlled substance.

John Smith, MD
1234 Medical Drive
San Antonio, TX 78231

Phone: 210-555-1234   **Fax:** 210-555-1235

Patient name: _Sandra Cooper_   **Date:** _08/05/_

Address: _1987 Bamboo Trail San Antonio, TX 78231_

Ortho-TriCyclen

#3 months

1 tab po qd

Refills: _3_

Dr.'s signature: _John Smith, MD_   **DEA #:** _AS123456_

Drug name and strength:_____

Quantity:_____

Refills: _____

Patient's name:_____

Translate sig: _____

What is the day supply? _____

Is the DEA number valid? _____

Joan Miller, MD
1234 Medical Drive
San Antonio, TX 78231

Phone: 210-555-1234   **Fax:** 210-555-1235

Patient name: _Elizabeth Martinez_   **Date:** _08/05/_

Address: _345 Brentfield Road San Antonio, TX 78231_

Tylenol 500mg

#30

1 tab po q4-6 hours prn for ha

Refills: _2_

Dr.'s signature: _Joan Miller, MD_   **DEA #:** _AS123456_

Drug name and strength:_____

Quantity:_____

Refills: _____

Patient's name:_____

Translate sig: _____

What is the day supply? _____

Is the DEA number valid? _____

Joan Miller, MD
1234 Medical Drive
San Antonio, TX 78231

Phone: 210-555-1234   **Fax:** 210-555-1235

Patient name: _Mark Anderson_   **Date:** _08/05/_

Address: _987 Swan Lake San Antonio, TX 78231_

Darvocet N-100

#40

1 tab po q 4-6 hours prn pain

Refills: _0_

Dr.'s signature: _Joan Miller, MD_   **DEA #:** _AS123456_

Drug name and strength:_____

Quantity: _____

Refills: _____

Patient's name:_____

Translate sig: _____

What is the day supply? _____

Is the DEA number valid? _____

DEA VERIFICATION ACTIVITY

Are the following DEA numbers valid?

1. AP137942
2. BR778931
3. BC263349
4. AS119844
5. BQ131582

6. AD459866
7. AT314219
8. BB244568
9. AM882693
10. BJ758137

WRITING PRESCRIPTIONS

Materials needed:

Prescription blanks

Reference sources such as *Drug Facts and Comparisons*, *PDR*, or the Internet

1. Using the reference sources, find the standard dosing for four different drugs, each in a different dosage form, and complete the worksheet below for each of the drugs.
2. Write a prescription for each drug, using the prescription blanks supplied by the instructor. Be sure to include all parts of the prescription, and write the directions using sig codes.

Drug #1 (tablet or capsule)

Drug name: _____

Standard dosing: _____

_____

Drug #2 (syrup, suspension, or elixir)

Drug name: _____

Standard dosing: _____

_____

Drug #3 (eye drop or ear drop)

Drug name: _____

Standard dosing: _____

_____

Drug #4 (nasal or oral inhaler)

Drug name: _____

Standard dosing: _____

_____

Assembly

Prescription Labels

On the next page is an example of a prescription label. Labels can be formatted in many different ways, but the information on them is always the same.

- **Vial label**: This is the label that is placed on the vial of medication that is given to the patient. This label must contain the following information:

    1. Pharmacy name, address, and phone number
    2. Prescription number
    3. Patient's name
    4. Fill date
    5. Drug name and strength
    6. Quantity
    7. Directions
    8. Doctor's name
    9. Refills
    10. Prescription expiration date

- **Prescription hardcopy label**: This label is placed on the back of the prescription hardcopy to be filed for recordkeeping. This label will have more information than the vial label; the example has the basic information typically found on a prescription hardcopy label.

- **Auxiliary labels**: Auxiliary labels are placed on vials to help the patient take their medication correctly. Examples of auxiliary labels include, "Take with food," "For topical use only," or "May cause drowsiness." Some labels will have an area for printing auxiliary labels.

- **Insurance signature log**: Insurance companies require signatures from the patient on all prescriptions. The signatures typically are on stickers that are placed into a log that can be audited by insurance companies.

- **Patient receipt**: This area has information such as prescription number, patient's name, drug name, strength, quantity, doctor's name, refills, and the cost of the prescription. There are two copies of the receipt, one for the patient's records and one to submit to the insurance company for manual claims.

- **Drug monograph**: This area has information about the drug, including brand name of drug, generic name, indication, side effects, how to take the medication, or what to do if a dose is missed.

Vial Label

Northwest Vista Pharmacy 3535 N. Ellison Drive San Antonio, TX 78231
210-353-7200

RX # 123456
Federico Lopez   6/30/
Allegra 180 mg Tablets   Qty: 30

Take 1 tablet by mouth daily.

Dr. Harry Hernandez
Refills: 3   Refillable until 10/30/08

Auxiliary Labels

Prescription Hardcopy Label

RX # 123456   Federico Lopez   DOB: 07/17/1974
Written: Allegra 180 mg   Written QTY: 30
Disp: Fexofenadine 180 mg   Written Date: 10/29/2007
NDC: 00088-1128-74   Exp Date: 10/30/2008
Ref Rem: 3   Ref Auth: 5
SIG: Take 1 tablet by mouth daily.

Dr. Belinda Padilla   DEA: AP9258134

Insurance Signature Log

Signature_____

Patient Receipt

Patient Receipt

Drug Monograph

8-Point Check

To assemble a prescription, a pharmacy technician needs a label, the original prescription, and the stock bottle. The technician verifies that the information on the label matches the information on the prescription. An 8-point check helps ensure that the prescription was typed correctly. The eight points or pieces of information are:

1. Patient's name (It is a good idea to check the patient's date of birth when checking the name to confirm that the medication is for the correct patient.)
2. Drug name
3. Drug strength
4. Quantity
5. Directions
6. Refills
7. Doctor's name
8. Written date

If any of these points do not match, then the prescription was typed incorrectly and must be corrected before continuing. In the following example, there is a prescription and the right portion of the label that prints out when you fill a prescription in RX Trainer.

Euell Crisp, MD
1214 Johnson Street, Suite 410
Alice, TX 78333

Phone: 210-655-1973   **Fax:** 210-655-1974

❶ Patient name: _Federico Lopez_   **❽ Date:** _10/29/_

Address: _210 South Tipton Freer, TX 78357_   **DOB:** _07/17/1974_

❷ _Allegra_   **❸** _180 mg_

❹ _#30_

❺ _1 tab po QD_

❻ Refills: _1_

❼ Dr.'s signature: _Euell Crisp, MD_   **DEA #:** _AC9258134_

RX #123456 **❶** Federico Lopez   **DOB:** 07/17/1974

Written: **❷** Allegra **❸** 180 mg   **Written QTY:** **❹** 30

Disp: Fexofenadine 180 mg*

NDC: 00088-1128-74

SIG: **❺** Take 1 tablet by mouth daily.

REF auth: **❻** 5   **REF rem:** 5

❼ Dr. Belinda Padilla   **DEA:** AP9258134

❽ Written date: 10/29/2007   **Exp date:** 10/30/2008

*The "Written" field and the "Disp" field do not match. Although the doctor wrote for Allegra 180 mg, the pharmacy will give the patient the generic form, Fexofenadine 180 mg. If the doctor does not want the pharmacy to dispense the generic to the patient, the doctor must write "Brand name medically necessary" on the prescription, and the pharmacy will dispense the brand-name medication. The patient may also request the brand over the generic, although the cost or copay for the patient may be higher.

After completing the 8-point check, verify that the correct stock bottle was pulled from the shelf before counting. You will match the National Drug Code (NDC) number on the stock bottle to the NDC number on the prescription hardcopy label. The NDC number uniquely identifies every drug on the market and is printed on the stock bottle's label. The NDC consists of three parts, as shown in this sample:

12345-	1234-	12
Manuf	Drug	Pkg

The first five digits represent the manufacturer. The next four digits represent the drug. The last two digits represent the package size. Once the technician verifies that the NDC number on the prescription hardcopy label matches the NDC number on the stock bottle's label, the technician is ready to count.

8-POINT CHECK ACTIVITY

Perform an 8-point check on the following prescriptions and labels. Each set has 3 errors; circle the errors on the label.

Belinda Padilla, MD
14087 O'Connor Road, Suite 600
San Antonio, TX 78247

Phone: 210-655-1973   **Fax:** 210-655-1974

Patient name: _Marissa Reynolds_   **Date:** _03/18/_

Address: _17928 Expedition Creek San Antonio, TX 78254_

Topamax 100mg

_#120_

2 tabs po am & 2 tabs hs

Refills: _5_

Dr.'s signature: _Belinda Padilla, MD_   **DEA #:** _BP7823591_

RX #123456 Marissa Reynolds   **DOB:** 11/13/1979

Written: Topamax 100mg   **Written QTY:** 30

Disp: Topamax 100mg

NDC: 00123-6584-00

SIG: Take 1 tablet by mouth in the morning and 2 tablets at bedtime.

REF auth: 6   **REF rem:** 6

Dr. Benjamin Padilla   **DEA:** BP7567917

Written date: 03/18/08   **Exp date:** 03/17/09

Joshua Gamboa, MD
103 Blueridge
San Antonio, TX 78235

Phone: 210-379-5702   **Fax:** 210-226-2737

Patient name: _Maria Arrellano_   **Date:** _02/21/_

Address: _103 Blueridge San Antonio, TX 78254_   **DOB:** _12/12/1986_

Nasonex 50mcg Nasal Spray

#1 unit

2 sprays/nostril qd

Refills: _0_

Dr.'s signature: _Joshua Gamboa, MD_   **DEA #:** _AG7632483_

RX #1234567 Maria Arevalo   **DOB:** 10/23/1969

Written: Nasonex 150 mg   **Written QTY:** 1 Unit

Dispensed: Nasonex 150 mg

NDC: 04513-2020-16

SIG: Use 2 sprays in each nostril once daily.

REF auth: 0   **REF rem:** 0

Dr. Joshua Gamboa   **DEA:** AG7632483

Written date: 07/08/08   **Exp date:** 07/07/09

John Nevada, MD
1069 South Pole Street
San Antonio, TX 78247

Phone: 210-291-0113   **Fax:** 210-291-0115

Patient name: _Sally Smith_ _____ **Date:** _02/29/_

Address: _109 North Parkway San Antonio, TX 78254_ **DOB:** _12/18/1981_

Ortho Evra

#9

1 patch weekly X 3 weeks then off for 1 week

Refills: _0_

Dr.'s signature: _John Nevada, MD_ _____ **DEA #:** _BP7823591_

RX #1234567 Sally Smith   **DOB:** 12/18/1981

Written: Ortho Evra Patch   **Written QTY:** 9 Patches

Dispensed: Ortho Evra Patch

NDC: 15957-3876-09

SIG: Apply 1 patch weekly for 3 weeks.

REF auth: 2   **REF rem:** 2

Dr. John Navajo   **DEA:** AN19831091

Written date: 07/08/08   **Exp date:** 07/07/09

Counting

Pharmacies typically use counting machines, digital scales, or automated dispensing machines; some may use a counting tray and a spatula to count out medications. A counting tray is made of hard plastic and has a flat area where the medication is counted, a spout on the upper-right corner, and a covered trench along the left side of the tray. The trench on the left side has an opening at the bottom that is used to pour the counted medication into a vial.

Before counting, use a paper towel and alcohol to ensure the tray and spatula are clean and free of residue from medications previously counted in the tray. To start counting, pour some of the tablets or capsules onto the flat counting area, lift the trench cover, and use a spatula to move the tablets or capsules into the trench in groups of five. When you have reached the number of tablets or capsules needed to fill the prescription, close the trench cover and pour any extra tablets or capsules back into the stock bottle, using the spout on the upper-right corner of the tray. Then use the opening at the bottom of the trench on the left side of the tray to pour the counted tablets or capsules into a vial.

Labeling and Auxiliary Labels

Placing a label on a vial of counted medication is fairly simple; there are just a few things to remember.

1. Always place the label on the vial as straight as possible.
2. Never use a torn label. If the label tears, reprint it.
3. Make sure the print is clear. If the print is too light, replenish the ink or toner in the printer and reprint the label.

Neatness and appearance are important in the pharmacy profession in order to earn and keep patients' trust. A prescription that is difficult to read or sloppy will affect the patient's perception of the pharmacy.

There may be auxiliary labels that should be placed on the vial in addition to the vial label. Auxiliary labels provide additional information to help the patient take medications correctly and safely; examples include "Take With Food," or "May Cause Drowsiness." The pharmacy technician may be expected to know which auxiliary labels should be used with different medications.

You now know all of the steps to filling a prescription, from taking in the prescription from the patient to counting and labeling. Practice by typing prescriptions into the RX Trainer software, printing labels, and counting medications. Verify each other's work. The instructor can act as the pharmacist and perform the final check.

Exceptions

Refill Requests

When a patient runs out of refills, the pharmacy can contact the patient's doctor for a refill approval. On the following page is a sample of a refill request form. Refill request forms can be formatted in many different ways, but the basic information will be the same on all of them.

Training Pharmacy
3001 Appletree Boulevard
San Antonio, TX 78251
Phone: 210-559-9987 Fax: 210-559-9988

REFILL REQUEST FORM

Dr.: Calvin Robins

Phone: 493-555-8000 Fax: 493-555-8001

Rx#: 10027

Patient name: Tommy DiVito

DOB: 02/21/1943

Medication: Actos 30mg

Qty: 30

Sig: Take 1 tablet by mouth daily.

Written date: 07/20/2007 Last filled: 05/01/2008

Pharmacy comments: _____

_____

Approved by: _____

Refused by: _____ Date: _____

Refills authorized: 1   2   3   4   5 ____ PRN

Physician comments: _____

_____

Information that appears on a refill request includes:

1. The pharmacy's name, address, and phone number
2. The doctor's name, phone number, and fax number if available
3. Prescription number (used by the pharmacy for tracking and recordkeeping)
4. The patient's name and date of birth
5. Drug name and strength
6. Quantity
7. Directions
8. Written date and last-filled date
9. An area for pharmacy comments
10. An area for the doctor's office to approve or deny refills and to make comments

The pharmacy may make comments that verify directions, note that the patient needs an early refill, or note insurance rejections, such as when the drug is not on the insurance company's formulary. The doctor's comments may include notes that the patient needs an appointment for further refills or that the prescription must last a certain length of time (e.g., 30 days).

The refill request form can be faxed to the doctor's office if they accept faxes, or the technician may call the doctor's office directly. The technician may have to leave a voice message on a refill line. Here is an example of a refill request from a pharmacy left on a doctor's refill line.

> **Pharmacy technician:** *This is Freddy with Training Pharmacy. I am calling for a refill approval on patient Tommy DiVito, date of birth 02/21/1943. Mr DiVito needs a refill on his Actos 30 mg tablets, quantity of 30. The directions are take one tablet by mouth daily. Last filled date was 05/01/2008. The pharmacy's number is 210-559-9987. Thank you.*

If you speak to someone at the doctor's office, you will still give the same information. Notice that the message does not include the prescription number or the written date. The pharmacy uses the prescription number for tracking and recordkeeping purposes. When refills are approved, it is considered a new prescription. Approved refills are not added to the old prescription, but there is a link between the new prescription and the old prescription number to keep track of the prescription. In addition, it is not necessary to give the written date of the prescription, because the doctor wrote the prescription and the doctor's office already has that information.

After faxing or calling on a refill request form, the technician will file it until the doctor's office calls and approves it. Some pharmacies file the forms in a specific location or box. When the doctor's office calls back, the technician notes the name of the person calling to approve or refuse the refills, the date, the number of refills approved, and any comments.

COMPLETING A REFILL REQUEST FORM

Make up information to fill in the blank refill request form. Pair up with a partner and take turns acting as the pharmacy and the doctor's office and practice calling in a refill request. Make sure that your partner gives all of the necessary information and uses proper telephone etiquette. If your instructor allows, you can use your cell phones to call your partner in order to get a realistic experience. If two rooms are available, one room can be used as the pharmacy and the other can be used as the doctor's office, and students can use cell phones to simulate refill request calls.

Training Pharmacy
3001 Appletree Boulevard
San Antonio, TX 78251
Phone: 210-559-9987 Fax: 210-559-9988

REFILL REQUEST FORM

Dr.: _____

Phone: _____ Fax: _____

Rx#: _____

Patient name: _____

DOB: _____

Medication: _____

Qty: _____

Sig: _____

Written date: _____ Last filled: _____

Pharmacy comments: _____

_____

Approved by: _____

Refused by: _____ Date: _____

Refills authorized: 1   2   3   4   5 _____ PRN

Physician comments: _____

_____

Prescription Transfers

Patients sometimes transfer their prescriptions from one pharmacy to another (for example, because the patient has moved or is visiting from out of town). If the patient is transferring prescriptions between two pharmacies in the same chain, for example, from one Walgreens to another, the transfer may be done electronically. If the patient is transferring prescriptions to a different chain, for example, from Walgreens to CVS, the pharmacist will have to call and get all of the information. Keep in mind that prescriptions for controlled substances can only be transferred one time; it is important to make the patient aware of this if the prescription has more than one refill available. Some states do not allow the transfer of certain medications, especially controlled medications, from out of state. In order to transfer a prescription, the patient must provide the following information:

1. Patient name
2. Date of birth
3. Name and phone number of the original pharmacy
4. Name of medication

The more information the technician has, the easier the transfer will be. The sample transfer form lists all of the information needed to complete the transfer. The patient only needs to provide the information listed above; the rest of the information on the form can be given by the pharmacy from which the prescription is being transferred.

Training Pharmacy
3001 Appletree Boulevard
San Antonio, TX 78251
Phone: 210-559-9987 Fax: 210-559-9988

Transferred from:

Pharmacy name: _____

Pharmacist name: _____

Address: _____

Phone number: _____

Pharmacy DEA #: _____

Patient information:

Name: _____

Address: _____

Phone number: _____

DOB: _____

Gender: _____

Allergies: _____

Insurance number: _____

Drug information:

Name: _____

Strength: _____

Quantity: _____

Rx #: _____

Date of original Rx: _____

Date of last refill: _____

Number of remaining refills: _____

Number of refills authorized: _____

Physician name: _____

Phone number: _____

DEA#: _____

Sig: _____

Insurance Cards

Prescription insurance coverage is a very big part of retail pharmacy and it is important for the pharmacy technician to be able to gather the information needed from the patient's insurance card. Each insurance card can look different, but the necessary information will be the same.

- **Bank identification number (BIN)**: This number identifies the insurance company that is going to pay the claim.

- **Processor control number (PCN)**: This number identifies the company that processes the claims for the insurance company. Each processor may handle multiple insurance companies. The processor control number can be all letters, all numbers, or a combination.

- **Member identification number**: This number identifies the member. It may be all letters, all numbers, or a combination.

- **Group number**: This number identifies the company for whom the member works and is used by the processor to adjudicate the claim.

INSURANCE CARD ACTIVITY

Materials needed:

Paper
Markers or colored pencils

The instructor assigns students to groups, and each group designs its own insurance card. Be sure to include all necessary information. Be creative and have fun deciding on your insurance company's name and logo.

Insurance Rejections

REJECT: Duplicate Paid/Captured Claim

Reason for reject: Prescription was filled today or yesterday at this pharmacy.
Solution: If this is a new prescription, log it in the computer. If this is a refill, void the refill and inform the patient the prescription is already filled.

Reason for reject: Prescription was filled at another pharmacy.
Solution: Inform the patient the prescription was filled at another pharmacy. Ask the patient if he or she would like to pick it up at the pharmacy where it was filled or transfer the prescription to your pharmacy.

Reason for reject: Patient took prescription to another pharmacy. The other pharmacy submitted the claim but did not have the medication in stock. The patient took back the prescription and brought it to your pharmacy. When you try to submit the claim, you discover the other pharmacy has not reversed the original claim.
Solution: Contact the other pharmacy and ask them to reverse the claim.

REJECT: Refill Too Soon

Reason for reject: Patient is unaware it is too soon to fill the prescription.
Solution: Inform the patient it is too soon to fill the prescription and give the patient the earliest date that his or her insurance will cover the medication.

Reason for reject: Patient is going out of town and will run out of medication before returning.
Solution: Call the insurance company for a vacation override. Depending on the patient's insurance plan, a vacation override may not be available. If a vacation override is not available, the patient may have

the option of transferring the prescription to a pharmacy in the city he or she is visiting. Transferring a prescription may not be possible if the patient is traveling out of the country or if the prescription is for a controlled medication. (In the case of a controlled medication, the doctor's office would also have to be called.) As a last resort, the patient may pay the full price for the medication out of pocket and submit manual claims to the insurance company.

Reason for reject: Patient has lost the medication, or it was stolen.
Solution: Call the insurance company for a lost or stolen override. Most insurance plans do not provide a lost or stolen override, and the patient will have to go without their medication or pay full price for the medication out of pocket.

Reason for reject: Dosage has changed.
Solution: If the doctor has told the patient to increase the dose, contact the doctor's office for a new prescription reflecting the new directions and quantity. After the pharmacy obtains the new prescription from the doctor's officer contact the insurance company for a change in dose override.

REJECT: Non-Formulary Drug/NDC Not Covered

Reason for reject: A non-formulary drug reject means the drug is not on the insurance company's list of covered medications. The insurance company may reject the claim altogether or may charge the patient a very high copay. This type of reject will usually return a list of alternate medications that are on the formulary. For example, an insurance may reject Prevacid and suggest Zantac, Pepcid, or Tagamet.
Solution: First, inform the patient that the medication is not on the insurance company's formulary. Tell the patient how much the prescription will cost; the patient may pay decide to pay full price for the medication. If the patient does not want to pay full price, offer to contact the doctor to have the medication switched to one of the suggested formulary medications. Unless the pharmacy tells you otherwise, *always* ask the patient's permission to contact the doctor's office to have a medication switched. Remember that some patients will confuse the insurance refusing to cover a medication with the pharmacy refusing to fill a prescription.

REJECT: Non-Matched Card Holder

Reason for reject: ID number submitted on the claim does not match the ID number in the insurance company's computer.
Solution: Verify the cardholder's ID number. If it is correct, contact the insurance for assistance.

REJECT: Coverage Expired

Reason for reject: The patient's coverage has expired. This is very common at the beginning of the year, and many patients will not realize their insurance has changed.

Solution: If the patient insists that the coverage is still in effect, contact the insurance company for assistance. If the insurance company states the patient has no active coverage, the patient will have to contact the benefits coordinator.

REJECT: Non-Matched Prescriber

Reason for reject: The patient's insurance will only cover prescriptions written by his or her primary care physician (PCP). Prescriptions written by any other physician will not be covered unless it is a prescription written by an emergency room physician.

Solution: If the prescription is written by an emergency room physician, contact the insurance company for an override. Otherwise, contact the patient's PCP for the same prescription.

REJECT: Prior Authorization

Reason for reject: The insurance company requires the physician to contact the insurance company and explain the reason behind the treatment being prescribed. This type of reject usually involves medications that are expensive or medications that are being dosed higher than normal. For example, Celebrex 200 mg usually is dosed once daily, but it may be prescribed twice daily.

Solution: Inform the patient of the need for prior authorization and offer to contact the physician's office. Explain that the physician's office will have to contact the patient's insurance company and that the process could take a few days to a week. The physician's office may decide to change the prescription rather than deal with the insurance company. It is up to the insurance company to decide whether or not to cover the medication. The patient always has the option of paying full price for the medication.

Telephone Etiquette

Imagine yourself in the pharmacy. Customers are at the pick-up window, at the drop-off window, and at the drive-through; someone's infant is crying loudly in the lobby; the murmur of pharmacy operations as the automation systems work and printers generate label after label. On top of all of this, the phone rings incessantly.

The phone will ring in the middle of all pharmacy activities. This is not an interruption, but rather a part of the job that requires immediate attention. Telephone etiquette is an important part of pharmacy operations, and customers or patients on the phone cannot be ignored. The following guidelines can help pharmacy technicians decide what should and should not be done over the telephone.

Customers do not appreciate waiting on the other end of a ringing phone, not being greeted properly, or being transferred from person to person several times in one telephone call. It is good practice for pharmacy staff to answer the telephone promptly and identify themselves and the pharmacy upon answering the telephone. Always mention the pharmacy name and your name when answering the telephone. Greet customers with a friendly attitude. Try smiling while you speak. Be prepared to answer questions. Have resources available so that customers do not have to wait. Customers feel good knowing that competent technicians are working in the pharmacy where they receive their medications.

It is a good idea to get into the habit of addressing customers by name. This helps people feel comfortable and shows that the technician is attentive to the customer's needs. Never interrupt a customer, and listen so you do not miss important information. Record all required demographic information. Speak clearly. If you do not have the answer to a question, ask the pharmacist or find someone who does have the answer. Get back to the customer as soon as possible. If you have to transfer a customer, tell him or her why, ask for permission to do so, and provide the name or department, and, if possible, the telephone number, of the person to whom you are transferring the customer. Do not leave customers on hold for extended periods of time.

Here is a sample telephone conversation using proper telephone etiquette.

Technician: *Thank you for calling Sterile Solutions Pharmacy. This is Steve. How can I help you?*

Customer: *This is Mrs. Ida Brown and I need a refill on my blood pressure medicine.*

Technician: *I will be happy to help you with that Mrs. Brown, do you have the refill number?*

(Be sure to use the customer's name during the conversation. Never use the customer's first name unless you are personally acquainted with the customer and you would normally use the person's first name. You can also address the customer as Ma'am or Sir; this is particularly helpful if the customer's name is hard to pronounce.)

Customer: *I'm sorry I don't have my bottle with me.*

Technician: *Not a problem Mrs. Brown, I just need to look up your profile. What is your date of birth?*

Customer: *Why do you need to know how old I am?*

(Some customers may be offended when asked for personal information. Explain politely why the information is necessary.)

Technician: *I'm sorry Mrs. Brown, I need your date of birth so that I can be sure I am looking at the right profile and fill the right medication for you.*

Customer: *May 3, 1955.*

Technician: *Thank you. What medication do you want to refill?*

Customer: *I need my lisinopril.*

Technician: *OK, Mrs. Brown, when would you like to pick up your refill?*

Customer: *I would like to pick it up this evening around 6 pm.*

Technician: *Let me check to make sure I have the medication in stock. May I put you on hold?*

(When putting a customer on hold, be sure to ask for the customer's permission and wait for a response. Some technicians automatically put a customer on hold without waiting for the customer's permission, which can make the customer angry. Never leave a customer on hold for too long, always check back with the customer if the information you are looking for is taking longer to find than you expected. Always give the customer the option of continuing to hold or offering to call the customer back when you find the information.)

Customer: *Yes.*

(When returning to the call, thank the customer for holding.)

Technician: *Thank you for holding Mrs. Brown. I do have the medication in stock and we will have it ready for you by 6 pm. Is there anything else I can do for you?*

Customer: *No, that's it, thank you.*

Technician: *Thank you, Mrs. Brown.*

Although it may seem funny to respond to the patient's "thank you" with a "thank you" instead of "you're welcome," always remember that without customers, there are no jobs as pharmacy technicians.

TELEPHONE ETIQUETTE ACTIVITY

Form into groups for this activity. The instructor will assign each group one of the following scenarios. Each group should imagine a dialogue that might occur between the technician and the individual who calls. Once the group writes down the dialogue, pick two people from the group to act the scene out in class. Remember that these are real situations pharmacy technicians will encounter on the job, and practice now will help performance later.

- Patient calls for refill and drug pharmacy is out of stock.

- Nurse calls to ask when the last time a prescription was filled for a patient.

- Angry patient calls and states the pharmacy gave wrong medication.

- Patient calls for a price check on a drug.

- Patient calls to find out if new prescription is ready.

- Patient calls to find out if doctor has approved refills.

- Another pharmacy calls to see if you have a drug in stock.

WORKING HOSPITAL PHARMACY

III

Medication Administration Record

The medication administration record (MAR) is generated from the medication order that the doctor sends to the pharmacy. The doctor's order always includes the schedule for the administration of drugs, the exact dosage form of the drug (tablet, capsule, solution, suspension, etc., rather than just "liquid"), the dosage strength, directions for use where appropriate, and route of administration. Transcribe the orders onto the MAR. Some doctors and nurses do not include all of the information needed; double check the work to make sure the prescription is filled correctly.

The pharmacy generates the MAR; it serves as a record of medication administration by the nursing staff. The MAR contains a list of the drugs dispensed from the pharmacy, the time of dispensing, the initials of the person dispensing, as well as the dosages and times of administration.

Instead of giving a set of dosage instructions (i.e., sig) with each drug, the MAR puts the medication order within a specific dosing schedule. This schedule tells when the medications are to be given to the patient and is normally determined by the institution. The times of administration may be listed across the top of a MAR according to a 24-hour clock. The nurse administering the medication may place a mark in the block underneath the time that the medication was administered to the patient. There may be blank spaces next to the time of administration to permit the pharmacy technician to note the time he or she dispensed the drugs or to initial the record. The nurse also initials the actual time of administration.

This is a sample MAR for patient Monica McDaniel. On a separate sheet of paper write down all the abbreviated terms and translate them. (For example, NKA means No Known Allergies.) Examine the drugs Monica received to determine the brand or generic names for the drugs, and translate the sig codes.

Medication Administration Record					
Patient name: Monica McDaniel 009887634 Diagnosis: Bipolar Disorder Doctor: Sandra Cooper			Allergies: NKA Ht: 5'9" Wt: 145 DOB: 8/7/1972		
Dates	**Medication-Dose Route of Adm.-Frequency**		**Administration**		
Start ⟋ Stop	Dosage/Direction/Amount		Date/Time/Initials		
	Mylanta 40cc po q6h prn				Pharmacy Use Only
	APAP 500mg ii tabs po q4h prn for HA and pain				Ok'd js
	Fluoxetine 20mg i cap po qd				Ok'd js
	Diazepam 4mg I tab po qd prn anxiety				Ok'd js
	MOM 30 cc po qam prn constipation				Ok'd js

Complete the blank MAR with a patient name, diagnosis, doctor, allergies, height, weight, date of birth, and seven drugs the patient is taking.

Medication Administration Record					
Patient name: Diagnosis: Doctor:			Allergies: Ht: Wt: DOB:		
Dates	**Medication-Dose Route of Adm.-Frequency**		**Administration**		
Start ⟋ Stop	Dosage/Direction/Amount		Date/Time/Initials		
					Pharmacy Use Only

Use the training software to type in the prescriptions under the inpatient prescriptions for your newly created patient. Be sure to create a new patient profile!

Formulary

A pharmacy's formulary is an important document, because it represents all of the drugs administered to patients. The Pharmacy and Therapeutics Committee chooses the drugs that make up the formulary. The committee has found that these drugs are the most effective for the patient population. The formulary should include information about how the drugs are used. Formularies should be updated often and published at least once a year. Updating the formulary ensures its effectiveness. Pharmacy technicians can sit in on the committee to understand why certain medications are not purchased and dispensed in the pharmacy. Complete the following activity and pretend that you are on the Pharmacy and Therapeutics Committee deciding what drugs to choose for your patients.

FORMULARY ACTIVITY

Create a formulary document for your classroom lab. Form into an even number of groups. Use the drugs in your pharmacy lab to create the formulary document. Categorize the drugs using the classifications below. The instructor can add more classifications and choose the number of drugs from each classification. To complete the formulary you will need the following information for each drug:

- Brand name
- Generic name
- NDC
- Manufacturer

Classifications of Drugs:

- Antibiotics
- Antivirals
- Antidepressants
- Antipsychotics
- Anticoagulants
- Pain medications (includes narcotics and non-narcotics)
- Diabetic medications
- Blood pressure medications

After each group has completed a list, input the formulary using the training software. You can create a formulary of drugs you frequently use in your training lab and prescriptions to go with them. This way you can practice filling prescriptions using drugs in your lab.

Unit Dosing

Pharmacy technicians prepare the unit-dose carts for inpatients each day. Much of the unit-dose work is done manually. Once a technician has filled the unit-dose orders the patient needs for a 24-hour period, the pharmacist checks them. The technician then delivers the medications to the patient floor or room number. Unit-dose carts can also be delivered to the nursing station at each ward, so that medications are ready for the nurse to administer to the patient when the dose is needed.

UNIT-DOSE–FILLING ACTIVITY

Fill the following patient unit doses with the appropriate medication and correct amount based upon the dosage for a 24-hour period. Use the Rx Trainer software to generate unit dose labels.

1. Crain, Isabelle　　(Rm) 121-3　　Filled by: _____
　　　　　　　　　　　　　　　　　Checked by: _____

　　　　　　　　　　　　　　　　　Quantity dispensed

　　Motrin 800 mg Q6H　　　　　　　_____
　　Dalmane 30 mg QD HS　　　　　　_____
　　Colace QD AM　　　　　　　　　_____

2. Robbins, Dave　　(Rm) 121-2　　Filled by: _____
　　　　　　　　　　　　　　　　　Checked by: _____

　　　　　　　　　　　　　　　　　Quantity dispensed

　　Metformin 800 mg Q4H　　　　　_____
　　Allopurinol 200 mg QD AM　　　　_____
　　Procardia 10 mg TID　　　　　　　_____

3. Dotzler, Susanna　　(Rm) 121-1　　Filled by: _____
　　　　　　　　　　　　　　　　　　Checked by: _____

　　　　　　　　　　　　　　　　　　Quantity dispensed

　　Lasix 40 mg QD AM　　　　　　　_____
　　Keflex 500 mg QID　　　　　　　　_____
　　Tenormin 100 mg Q12H　　　　　　_____

Sample label:

```
Drug: LASIX 40mg
NDC: 12345-1234-12
Manufacturer: Abbott Laboratories
Lot #: 123AB45
Exp. date: 10/31/2010
RPh:_____Tech:_____
```

Intravenous Lab

The most critical patients for whom pharmacies prepare medications are patients who are receiving intravenous (IV) therapy. Pharmacy technicians need to be very careful when preparing IV medications. Every caution must be taken in order to avoid contaminating medication and ultimately the patient. The IV route is the most dangerous route of administration. This route is introduced directly into the bloodstream. An IV medication that is improperly prepared can cause serious consequences, including infections, emboli, occlusions, and even death.

Hand Washing

Hand washing is an essential part of practicing good aseptic technique. The environment and the technician must be free of any disease-causing microorganisms when technicians begin to make intravenous admixtures. Hand washing in the IV room requires a bit more than rubbing your hands together under the faucet for a few seconds. Use the following checklist as a guide for proper hand washing technique.

Hand Washing Checklist

✓ Gather needed supplies: sink, liquid soap, nail pick, nail scrub, and paper towels.

✓ Remove all jewelry.

✓ Adjust water temperature. It should be lukewarm. Remember: no splashing!

✓ Open the scrub brush.

✓ Wet hands and make sure to apply plenty of soap.

✓ Clean fingernails with pick.

✓ Begin scrubbing hands in circular motions, working up from hands to elbows.

✓ Rinse soap from hands to elbows until soap is gone.

✓ Use paper towel without touching anything except clean towel, and pat dry from hands up to elbows.

✓ Use a paper towel to turn off water.

The first priority is to keep patients safe and help them get well; hand washing is one way to achieve that. It may be the most important thing a pharmacy technician can do to practice good aseptic technique. Practice these hand washing steps until they become second nature.

Horizontal and Vertical Laminar Flow Hoods

Laminar flow hoods are important because they keep the air in an IV room clean and free of dust particles. This equipment is essential to proper aseptic technique. Whether they are horizontal or vertical, the flow hoods provide clean air to the area where the technician is working. The constant air flow removes contaminants and provides a sterile environment. Use the following checklist as a guide for proper cleaning of the flow hood.

Flow Hood Cleaning Checklist

✓ Gather supplies: 4x4 gauze, 70% alcohol.

✓ The hood should be turned on if it has been off; allow it to run for at least 30 minutes.

✓ Start by cleaning the IV pole and IV hooks with a damp alcohol gauze.

✓ Next clean the right side of the flow hood, beginning at the back. Use a damp alcohol gauze and clean up and down from top to bottom in overlapping strokes.

✓ Next clean the left side of the flow hood, beginning at the back. Use a damp alcohol gauze and clean up and down from top to bottom in overlapping strokes.

✓ In a horizontal laminar flow hood, clean the floor or work surface last. Start at the back of the floor and clean from side to side until you reach the front. With a vertical flow hood, clean the floor before cleaning the glass shield. Clean the glass shield last.

✓ Dispose of the alcohol gauze properly.

Needles and Syringes

Pharmacy technicians must use aseptic technique when using needles and syringes. Using this technique will minimize injury and contamination. The parts of the needle include the following:

- Bevel tip
- Bevel
- Bevel heel
- Shaft
- Hub

Needles are supplied in many sizes. It is important for technicians to become familiar with two numbers describing the needle size: the gauge of the needle and the length of the needle. The gauge relates to the diameter of the bore, which is how big around it is in the shaft. A rule of thumb for technicians to remember is that the bigger the gauge, the smaller the bore. The length of a needle shaft is measured in inches and ranges from ⅜ to 3 inches.

Needles come individually wrapped and should remain that way until just before use. When using needles for compounding, no part of the needle should be touched. The needle should remain sterile.

There are multiple types of needles. For example, a filter needle is used when removing liquid drug from a glass ampule. The filter needle filters out any glass that was broken into the liquid and prevents it from being injected into the patient.

Needles are attached to syringes, which are made of either glass or plastic. Some medications react with plastic and could effect potency and stability; glass syringes are necessary in these cases. Except for those uses, most pharmacies will carry plastic syringes because they are inexpensive and durable. The parts of the syringe include the following:

- Flat end
- Plunger
- Top collar
- Plunger piston
- Barrel
- Calibration marks
- Luer lock tip

The luer lock secures the needle with the syringe. Be aware that some needles do not have this lock and are held together by friction. Syringe sizes range from 1 ml to 60 ml. A rule of thumb is the greater the syringe capacity, the greater the interval of calibration lines. In an ideal situation, the volume of liquid should take up no more than two thirds of the syringe capacity. When measuring the drug solution, line up the final edge of the plunger piston to the calibration mark desired. Syringes are individually wrapped and should remain that way until use. The luer lock or the plunger that travels in and out of the barrel should not be touched and should remain sterile. Make sure to choose the correct syringe and needle combination. The following is a good guide:

- 3 ml or 5 ml syringes use a 20-gauge needle

- 10 ml or 20 ml syringes use an 18-gauge needle

When using glass ampules, use a filter needle first, then change to a regular needle. A larger needle may result in coring, which occurs when the insertion of the needle into the rubber stopper of a vial slices a piece of that rubber and it falls into the liquid drug. The instructor can demonstrate the non-coring method of inserting the syringe.

Air bubbles must be removed from syringes. Air bubbles can compromise the accuracy of measurement. To remove air bubbles, firmly hold the syringe in a vertical position, pull the plunger back slightly, use the knuckles to tap the bubbles out, pull the plunger down slightly again, then push the plunger up until the liquid fully primes the needle.

Be sure to dispose of needles and syringes according to the institutional policies of the employer. Usually needles are discarded in puncture-resistant containers called *sharps containers*. Most hospitals or compounding pharmacies have policies and procedures on recapping needles as required by the Occupational Safety and Health Administration (OSHA). The one-handed scoop method is most common. This is accomplished by positioning the cap on the laminar hood surface and aiming the needle inside through a scooping method. Once the cap is scooped on, the technician can shut it with the other hand. Be sure to report any needle sticks to a supervisor and complete any required documentation.

Needle and Syringe Checklist

✓ Position needle and syringe packages 6 inches into the hood.

✓ Open needle packaging and peel back like a banana.

✓ Hold the needle in one hand facing the back of the hood so that airflow surrounds the needle.

✓ Open the syringe packaging and peel back like a banana.

✓ Hold syringe by barrel only and angle barrel tip toward the back of the hood so that airflow surrounds the needle.

✓ Connect the needle to the syringe, but do not block airflow.

✓ Discard wraps in waste container beside the laminar flow hood workstation.

✓ After use of needle and syringe, recap needle using the one-handed scoop method.

✓ Wait for pharmacist check.

✓ Dispose capped needles in the sharps container.

Ampules Checklist

✓ Gather supplies: 1 ampule, needle, syringe, a 100 ml IV bag, and alcohol swabs.

✓ Place supplies into the laminar flow hood to maximize airflow.

✓ Using proper aseptic technique, open the syringe and filter needle and attach them together.

✓ Remove liquid from the top of the ampule by using a flicking motion.

✓ Wipe the neck of the ampule with an alcohol swab, holding it between the index finger and the thumb. Break the top off at a 20° angle.

✓ Make sure there is no air in the syringe and insert the needle into the ampule. Be sure to draw the plunger back quickly and with maximum control.

✓ Remove the filter needle and recap, using the one-handed scoop method.

✓ Attach a regular needle and wait for the pharmacist to check.

✓ After the pharmacist checks the syringe and drug used, inject the solution into the IV bag.

✓ Place label onto the IV bag.

✓ Discard needle in the sharps container.

✓ Discard other materials in a regular trash receptacle.

Vials Checklist

✓ Gather supplies: liquid vial, needle, syringe, 100 ml IV bag, and alcohol swabs.

✓ Place supplies into the laminar flow hood to maximize airflow.

✓ Using proper aseptic technique, open the syringe and needle and attach them together.

✓ Remove the plastic cap from the top of the vial and set off to the side.

✓ Use an alcohol swab to wipe the rubber stopper in one motion three times.

✓ Pick up the syringe and pull plunger back to desired amount of solution.

✓ Insert needle into vial using the non-coring technique.

✓ Push the air into the vial and practice using the milking method to withdraw the amount of solution needed.

✓ After the pharmacist checks the syringe and drug used, inject the solution into the IV bag.

✓ Place label onto IV bag.

✓ Discard needle in the sharps container.

✓ Discard other materials in a regular trash receptacle.

Reconstituting Checklist

✓ Gather supplies: liquid vial, powdered vial, needle, syringe, 100 ml IV bag, and alcohol swabs.

✓ Place supplies into the laminar flow hood to maximize airflow.

✓ Using proper aseptic technique, open the syringe and needle and attach them together.

✓ Remove the plastic cap from the top of the vial and set off to the side.

✓ Use an alcohol swab to wipe the rubber stopper in one motion three times.

✓ Pick up the syringe and pull plunger back to desired amount of solution.

✓ Insert needle into vial using the non-coring technique.

✓ Push the air into the vial and practice using the milking method to withdraw the amount of solution needed.

✓ Inject liquid into the powdered vial, remove syringe, and allow medication to dissolve.

✓ Reinsert needle into reconstituted vial and remove the desired amount of drug.

✓ After the pharmacist checks the syringe and drug used, inject the solution into the IV bag.

✓ Place label onto the IV bag.

✓ Discard needle in the sharps container.

✓ Discard other materials in regular trash receptacle.

Preparation of Chemotherapy IVs

Pharmacy technicians are responsible for preparing chemotherapy intravenous solutions. Although aseptic technique is used when preparing chemotherapy solutions, there are a few differences when working with these hazardous drugs.

Technicians must use a vertical laminar flow hood when preparing chemotherapy intravenous solutions. In a vertical laminar flow hood, the air is blown in a downward motion. This flow hood has a glass shield and it is used to protect the pharmacy technician from the chemotherapy drug in the case of spills or splashes. Spill kits should be available nearby, and if a spill occurs, the area should be cleaned three times. When preparing chemotherapy drugs, technicians must wear protective clothing such as:

• Protective non-absorbent gown with cuffs

• Two pairs of gloves

• Face mask

• Shoe covers

• Hair cover

When preparing chemotherapy vials the technician must remember to vent each vial to reduce spraying. Remember to clean surfaces of all materials used with alcohol swabs. Label each intravenous bag as hazardous or chemotherapy and dispose of chemotherapy drugs according to institutional policy.

Chemotherapy Preparation Checklist

✓ Wash hands and dress in protective clothing.

✓ Cover flow hood surface with a plastic absorbent paper.

✓ Clean hood with 70% isopropyl alcohol.

✓ Place supplies in flow hood.

✓ Clean all supply surfaces with alcohol swabs.

✓ Perform all manipulations with vials, solutions, or ampules using aseptic technique. (Remember airflow is blowing down.)

✓ Place all chemotherapy needles and syringes in a chemotherapy sharps container.

✓ Label all intravenous bags with required information.

✓ Wait for a pharmacist check.

✓ Dispose of all chemotherapy drug supplies in a designated container according to institutional policy.

Small- and Large-Volume Parenterals

When compounding drugs using aseptic technique, a common method is to add the drug into a small-volume parenteral (SVP), also known as a piggyback, which is any solution that is less than or equal to 100 ml. Large-volume parenterals (LVP) are IV solutions greater than 100 ml in volume. LVPs are solutions like dextrose or sodium chloride that are sometimes used as continuous infusions or used for intermittent infusions. Pharmacy technicians will add drug additives to both SVPs and LVPs.

Total Parenteral Nutrition

Total parenteral nutrition (TPN) used to be known as *hyperalimentation*. This type of IV includes all nutrients needed to sustain a patient's life. TPNs contain fats, water, electrolytes, vitamin, carbohydrates, protein, and trace elements. TPN is used for patients who cannot eat or are in a coma.

Procedures for dispensing TPNs vary from institution to institution. Great care must be taken when dispensing a TPN, because the potential for mistakes is high and serious injury to a patient can occur. The pharmacist should verify all TPN calculations and the solutions and ingredients. Quality control procedures need to be followed and measured in order to ensure safety.

Labeling Intravenous Drugs

United States Pharmacopeia's (USP) 797 introduced new minimum labeling standards for compounding sterile preparations. The following is a sample label:

Cefazolin	1 gm
In 10% dextrose in water	50 ml
Total volume	250 ml
Infuse intravenously over 30 min. every 6 hours	
Ancef	
Use before: 1600 3/2/09	
Prepared by: CEM	Checked by: TKO
Keep refrigerated.	

Labels should be typed or electronically printed in a standard format. This will ensure legibility and help prevent errors. Use the metric system instead of the apothecary system to measure. In the pharmacy, only a licensed pharmacist or authorized pharmacy technician can label and dispense medications.

The label above includes the name of the drug in generic and brand name to reduce errors. The names and strengths of all products used to compound the drug should be listed. The total volume is expressed in the metric system. The beyond-use date is the last date that the sterile preparation can be used by the patient. Storage instructions (such as refrigeration requirements) can be placed directly on to the label or added as an auxiliary label. Initial your work!

Labels that are delivered to specific patients must have patient information on them. The following is a sample label used in an institutional or home health care setting:

Training Pharmacy Hospital	
Christina Prosser	E 1123
883778-0034	Bag # 2
Time due: 1800 31 May 09	
Vancomycin	500 mg
NaCl 0.9%	150 ml
Total volume	150 ml
Infuse intravenously over 90 min. every 8 hours	
Prepared by: CEM	Checked by: TKO
Use before: 2300 6 June 09	

Auxiliary labels provide supplemental information or instructions. Technicians use these because the space on the regular label is limited. This information is placed next to the regular label on a container and is highlighted in different colors for easy reading. Examples of some auxiliary labels include, "Protect from light," "Refrigerate," "Do not shake," "Shake well," and "For the eye."

Batching and Pre-Packing

Batching means to prepare a multiple set of drugs that will be needed in the future. Compounding the same drug preparation at one time is the process of batching. Labels are also needed for batches made in the pharmacy. The following is a batch label:

Amoxicillin   500 mg
Manufacturer name: SmithKline Beecham
Lot number: OHG6678
Expiration date: 02/10
Quantity: 30 capsules
Prepared by: CEM
Checked by: TKO

Practice generating labels and labeling training products in the lab setting using the software provided with this workbook.

SPECIAL TOPICS IN PHARMACY

IV

Ethics in Pharmacy: A Class Discussion

What does the word *ethics* mean? As a member of society, ethics generally means following a set of standards. These standards or values are considered normal for the community and become a guideline for all to follow. This practice is the same in many professions, including pharmacy. The standards in the pharmacy practice can be found in the form of laws. Establishing state boards of pharmacy for technicians was an important milestone in pharmacy history. Creating standards and laws has given a voice for the pharmacy technician and helps to keep technicians and patients safe.

So what does *ethics* mean to you as a technician? In addition to following the rules and guidelines of the profession, each technician also follows a personal set of values that guides his or her actions. Each of us is responsible for our decisions and choices.

Discuss the following scenarios. Ask yourself what the pharmacy technician should do in these cases.

Case One

You work as a technician in a retail chain pharmacy. You have been employed for nearly six months and, through rotating at different stores and attending company functions, you have made many technician friends. You have been spending a lot of time with Sofia Dabalsa, a technician at a neighboring pharmacy. You like her because you have a lot in common and enjoy talking about health care issues, new drugs, and topics in pharmacy. One day during lunch Sofia asks you if you have ever thought of selling Viagra. Jokingly you respond, "I do. I sell it every day at my pharmacy!" Sofia's serious expression lets you know that she means to sell it to someone other than a patient. Sofia proceeds to tell you that she has a friend who pays her $30 per Viagra pill. She has sold a bottle of 30 to him and made almost $1,000. This is just as much as she makes in two weeks. Sofia asks if you would be interested in partnering with her to take the Viagra from the pharmacy and sell it to her friend for extra cash.

- What are the ethical implications in this case?

- How would you respond to Sofia's request?

- Would you report it?

- If you do report it, who would you tell?

- If you do not report it, what might happen?

Case Two

Ben Jackson is a hardworking technician. He has received awards such as "employee of the month" and "technician of the year" for stellar performance in the pharmacy where he works. He is a father of three and recently has been having a tough time at home. Ben's wife asked for a divorce and wanted to move away to another state without the children. His wife moved away the week the divorce was finalized. Health insurance for Ben's family was obtained through his ex-wife's job, and he can't afford to get health coverage for himself or for the children for 45 days. Ben's son Jeremy comes down with a bad case of the flu. He has had these symptoms before, and last year the family doctor prescribed him some benadryl and amoxicillin capsules. Although he has no refills in his profile for these drugs, Ben decides to refill the prescriptions without having called the doctor. His rationale is that it will take too long and he does not have insurance. Because Ben works in the pharmacy and is an excellent technician, he knows how the computer database operates and covers his tracks. Ben fills the fake prescription amidst the busy day and stuffs the medication in his coat pocket when no one sees.

- What are the ethical implications in this case?

- Is this action justified?

- What would happen if Jeremy has an adverse reaction to the drugs?

- If you were Ben's supervisor and you caught him stealing these drugs, what would you do?

Pharmacy Technician Law: A Quick Guide

Pure Food and Drug Act of 1906

Prohibits interstate transportation or sale of adulterated drugs. Drugs did not need to be labeled but could not contain any false information about the strength or purity of the drug. This law was insufficient, and more legislation was eventually needed.

Food, Drug, and Cosmetic Act of 1938

Historical and most important law in pharmacy history because it created the Food and Drug Administration (FDA) and required manufacturers of new drugs to go through an application process before marketing them to the public. At this time drugs were to be safe for human consumption but were not required to be effective.

Durham-Humphrey Amendment

Drug containers were required to contain the following statement: "Caution: Federal law prohibits dispensing without prescription." This law differentiated between prescription drugs and over-the-counter drugs.

Kefauver-Harris Amendment

Expanded on the FDC Act of 1938 and required that drugs also be effective as well as safe for human consumption. Manufacturers must file an investigational new drug application with the FDA before conducting human clinical trials.

Comprehensive Drug Abuse Prevention and Control Act of 1970

Also known as the Controlled Substances Act and was created to control drug abuse. As a result of this legislation the Drug Enforcement Agency (DEA) was created. This act also classified drugs with high potential for abuse as controlled substances and ranked them into five schedules:

- **Schedule I**: highest potential for abuse with no medicinal purposes
- **Schedule II**: high potential for abuse
- **Schedule III**: moderate potential for abuse
- **Schedule IV**: low potential for abuse
- **Schedule V**: lowest potential for abuse

Poison Prevention and Packaging Act of 1970

Enacted in order to prevent accidental child poisoning from drugs. This act requires that OTC and legend drugs be packaged in child-resistant containers. By law, the elderly can request easy-open containers but must sign a waiver.

Drug Listing Act of 1972

FDA has the authority to compile a list of drugs currently on the market. Each drug is required to have a National Drug Code (NDC) number that identifies the manufacturer, drug formula, and size and type of packaging.

Drug Price Competition and Patent Term Restoration Act of 1984

This law encouraged production of both generic and brand name drugs. Less costly generic drugs with identical chemical composition can be substituted for the brand name drug in prescriptions.

Prescription Drug Marketing Act of 1987

This law prohibits reimportation of drugs into the United States as well as selling, trading, or distributing drug samples.

Omnibus Budget Reconciliation Act of 1990 (OBRA-90)

This law requires that each state establish standards for drug use review (DURs) by the pharmacists. Pharmacists must offer to counsel each patient and discuss their drug regimen.

Health Insurance Portability and Accountability Act of 1996 (HIPAA)

This law allows individuals to move health insurance from employer to employer without restrictions. This law also has introduced rules safeguarding patient confidentiality or records and conditions. Each pharmacy should provide a private area for consultations and provide training for employees. Technicians must not divulge any patient information outside of the pharmacy.

PHARMACY LAW ACTIVITY

Read the following scenarios and decide which law was violated. Write down the name of the law violated in the space provided.

Over the telephone, the technician discusses with the patient's husband what medication his wife received from her doctor.

_____

The technician does not clarify whether or not the patient needs easy-open caps and dispenses the wrong one.

_____

The pharmacist purchases drugs from an online store that are imported from China and sells them to customers.

_____

The pharmacist refuses to counsel a patient because the pharmacist is on lunch break.

_____

A manufacturing company decides to create a new drug and begins marketing to the public without FDA approval.

_____

A prescription drug is labeled without the statement: "Caution: Federal law prohibits dispensing without a prescription."

_____

This agency monitors drugs that are easily abused.

_____

Medication Errors

Medication errors can occur in a number of different ways. A technician may misread a prescription because the doctor's handwriting was illegible; a drug was placed in the incorrect location and dispensed in place of some other drug that has similar packaging. Every effort must be made to eliminate errors. The pharmacy technician's job includes double- and triple-checking the work of the technician and others. Be sure to ask the pharmacist for help if you need to clarify a prescription.

Remembering the patient's rights is important to minimizing medication errors. The patient's rights are:

- Right medication

- Right dose

- Right route

- Right time

- Right patient

Keep in mind the following when filling a prescription:

- Illegible doctor's writing should be interpreted by more than one person or confirmed with the doctor.

- Be aware of look-alike and sound-alike drugs and *never* guess.

- Clarify orders that are ambiguous, such as strengths, spacing, zeros, and decimal points.

- Use only the approved abbreviations.

- Use auxiliary labels to help patients understand the proper use of the drug dispensed.

- Follow the quality assurance program at the pharmacy.

MEDICATION ERRORS ONLINE ACTIVITY

Visit a search engine like google.com or yahoo.com on the Internet. Find an article or news story on medication errors. Print the article and bring it to class. Each student should summarize his or her article and discuss in class.

HIV: HOW MUCH DO YOU KNOW?

Take the following quiz to test your current knowledge. Decide if the statement is true or false.[1]

_____1. HIV is a disease that has no cure.

_____2. New drug treatments for HIV/AIDS have lowered the incidence of the disease in the United States.

_____3. Signs and symptoms of HIV/AIDS include loss of appetite, fever, rashes, lethargy, and lack of resistance to infections.

_____4. HIV is spread through hugging, touching, or kissing.

_____5. AIDS can be transmitted from sneezing or coughing.

_____6. Only drug users and gay men need to be tested for HIV/AIDS.

_____7. Women cannot get HIV if they use birth control pills.

_____8. People who are infected with HIV look different than everyone else.

_____9. People who have HIV and who inject drugs can pass HIV to another person using the same needle.

_____10. HIV is present in the blood, semen, breast milk, and vaginal secretions of people who are infected.

Scenarios

Discuss the following scenarios in class.

Scenario 1

Anthony works at a job where he is highly visible and works closely with customers. In the past couple of weeks there has been no serious change in his work performance but he has been looking ill. Anthony has lost a lot of weight and looks weak and frail. Every time you ask how he is doing he gets irritated and says, "I am fine!" and then changes the subject. He has began missing work due to doctor's appointments. You have heard through other workers that Anthony may have AIDS, and other workers complain about working with him.

- What are the legal implications involved in this situation?

- Can you ask Anthony to disclose any information?

- How would the employer address Anthony's coworkers' concerns?

1 *Quiz Answers:* 1. T; 2. T; 3. T; 4. F; 5. F; 6. F; 7. F; 8. F; 9. T; 10. T

Scenario 2

Jacqueline works for a major pharmaceutical company. She has been with this company for the past 10 years, and she has been promoted twice. Recently she disclosed to her employer that she has HIV. She asked that this information be kept confidential. Jacqueline has been in her current position for 3 years and continues to perform excellently, but since her disclosure, she has received disciplinary write-ups for poor work performance and tardiness. Last week upon arrival to her job she found that many of her job responsibilities had been reassigned to someone else. She was even given a desk in a remote location of the building. Jacqueline confronted her supervisor of these rather rapid changes and was informed that they were necessary to protect her coworkers.

- Can Jacqueline's employer take away her job responsibilities and move her desk?

- Does the employer have to honor her request about keeping her HIV status confidential?

Sexual Harassment on the Job

Sexual harassment occurs when anyone, male or female, expresses unwelcome sexual advances, requests sexual favors, or inappropriately verbalizes or touches another person in a sexual manner. It is sexual harassment when:

- The employee submits to the conduct as a condition of his or her employment.

- The employee rejects sexual conduct, and the rejection is used by the harasser as a basis for employment decisions affecting the employee.

- The employee's job performance is affected in a negative way due to inappropriate sexual conduct or because the work environment has become hostile.

Forms of Sexual Harassment

- Physical contact

  » Unwelcome hugging, sexual touching, or kissing

  » Pinching, grabbing, or patting inappropriately

  » Standing too close

  » Intentionally brushing against another person

  » Rape or attempted rape

  » Sexual assault or forced fondling

- Verbal conduct

  » Sexual jokes or lewd humor

  » Talking about how someone looks, especially about parts of the body

  » Catcalls, whistles, and name-calling (baby, honey, sexy)

  » Repeatedly asking someone out for a date

- Visual conduct

  » Pictures in work area of sexual material, pornographic material, or cartoons

  » Emails containing sexual material

  » Staring

  » Suggestive gestures or looks, licking of lips, or blowing kisses

The instructor may deliver a presentation to help future technicians better understand other aspects of sexual harassment. Many workplaces include training regarding sexual harassment.

Discrimination at Work

Discrimination unfortunately has many faces. Employees can be discriminated against because of race, color, national origin, age, religion, sexual preference, or sex. It is best to be informed about discrimination, because then you can better handle a situation that may arise.

It is illegal for any employer to make employment decisions based on an individual's race, color, or national origin. Any action taken by an employer that uses race, color, or national origin as requirement for the job is illegal and should be reported to the Equal Opportunity Office.

It is against the law for employers to discriminate on the basis of an individual's age. No person can be forced into retirement. Laws differ from state to state.

Failing to accommodate the religious practices of individuals is unlawful. This can include observing a sabbath or religious holidays. Employers need to show that a hardship would result from an employee's religious practices before refusing requests.

Sex discrimination protects both females and males. Most laws originated to protect women in the workplace and are still the main focus today. Sex discrimination can include separate lines of tenure or promotion and payment of different wages for the same work.

States provide protection to employees on each of the discriminatory categories, and some states or local jurisdictions may provide additional protections.

Answer the following questions:

- Have you been discriminated against at work or in any other situation?

- Has anyone you know ever been discriminated against?

- Did you receive any help to correct the situation?

- If not, what could have been done to correct the situation?

Activity Guidelines for Instructors

Split students into groups. Brainstorm some discrimination examples with students.

Some may include: name-calling, sexual advances, teasing, and derogatory names for sex or race. While you discuss each group's answers, purposely leave one group out of the discussion. Later you can discuss how that could be considered a form of discrimination. Maybe that group was too young, too old, all had blue eyes, or something in common to discriminate against.

Give examples of discrimination such as a pregnant woman who frequently leaves at midday, a gay male who is passed on for a promotion after disclosing his sexuality, or a 60-year-old obese female who does not move as fast as her younger coworkers. Ask the students to identify techniques used to confront discrimination at work.

APPENDIX

Prescription Samples

Use the following prescriptions to input into the online pharmacy. The more you practice, the better you will become at recognizing sig codes and controlled substances, creating patient profiles, learning what is required on the prescription, figuring day supply, and verifying DEA numbers.

John Smith, MD
1234 Medical Drive
San Antonio, TX 78231

Phone: 210-555-1234   **Fax:** 210-555-1235

Patient name: _Jane Doe_   **Date:** _08/05/_

Address: _123 Drury Lane San Antonio, TX 78231_

Amoxil 875mg

#30

1 tab po tid x 10 days

Refills: _0_

Dr.'s signature: _John Smith, MD_   **DEA #:** _AS123456_

Joan Miller, MD
1234 Medical Drive
Chicago, IL 44987

Phone: 210-532-0987   **Fax:** 210-525-9877

Patient name: *Joseph Fiennes*   **Date:** *08/05/*

Address: *209 Theater Avenue Chicago, IL 44987*

Lisinopril 20mg

#30

1 tab po qd

Refills: *6*

Dr.'s signature: *Joan Miller, MD*   **DEA #:** *AS123456*

Herbert Lewis, MD
3456 Pasteur Boulevard
Los Angeles, CA 90231

Phone: 908-222-0090   **Fax:** 908-222-0098

Patient name: _Michael Duncan_ _____ **Date:** _08/05/_

Address: _2988 Birch Trail Los Angeles, CA 90231_ _____

Lasix 40mg

_#30_

1 tab po qd

Refills: _1_

Dr.'s signature: _Herbert Lewis, MD_ _____ **DEA #:** _AS123456_

Robert Kelley, MD
8976 Mulberry Lane
San Antonio, TX 78231

Phone: 210-667-8975   **Fax:** 210-555-1235

Patient name: _Alicia Griffon_   **Date:** _08/05/_

Address: _3221 Justice Lane San Antonio, TX 78234_

Albuterol MDI

#1 unit

Inhale 1-2 puffs q4-6 hours prn

Refills: _3_

Dr.'s signature: _Robert Kelley, MD_   **DEA #:** _AS123456_

John Smith, MD
1234 Medical Drive
San Antonio, TX 78231

Phone: 210-555-1234   **Fax:** 210-555-1235

Patient name: _Angela Romero_   **Date:** _08/05/_

Address: _3765 Lilly Pond San Antonio, TX 78231_

Vicodin 500mg

_#20_

1 tab po q4-6 hours prn pain

Refills: _0_

Dr.'s signature: _John Smith, MD_   **DEA #:** _AS123456_

John Smith, MD
1234 Medical Drive
San Antonio, TX 78231

Phone: 210-555-1234   **Fax:** 210-555-1235

Patient name: _Sandra Cooper_   **Date:** _08/05/_

Address: _1987 Bamboo Trail San Antonio, TX 78231_

Ortho-TriCyclen

#3 months

1 tab po qd

Refills: _3_

Dr.'s signature: _John Smith, MD_   **DEA #:** _AS123456_

Joan Miller, MD
1234 Medical Drive
San Antonio, TX 78231

Phone: 210-555-1234   **Fax:** 210-555-1235

Patient name: _Elizabeth Martinez_   **Date:** _08/05/_
Address: _345 Brentfield Road San Antonio, TX 78231_

Tylenol 500mg

#30

1 tab po q4-6 hours prn for ha

Refills: _2_

Dr.'s signature: _Joan Miller, MD_   **DEA #:** _AS123456_

Joan Miller, MD
1234 Medical Drive
San Antonio, TX 78231

Phone: 210-555-1234   **Fax:** 210-555-1235

Patient name: _Mark Anderson_ _____**Date:** _08/05/_

Address: _9987 Swan Lake San Antonio, TX 78231_ _____

Darvocet N-100

#40

1 tab po q 4-6 hours prn pain

Refills: _0_

Dr.'s signature: _Joan Miller, MD_ _____ **DEA #:** _AS123456_

John Smith, MD
1234 Medical Drive
San Antonio, TX 78231

Phone: 210-555-1234   **Fax:** 210-555-1235

Patient name: _Lucy Balle_   **Date:** _08/05/_

Address: _118923 Candlewood Lane San Antonio, TX 78231_

Flonase NS

#1 unit

Spray 1 puff nasally bid

Refills: _3_

Dr.'s signature: _John Smith, MD_   **DEA #:** _AS123456_

John Smith, MD
1234 Medical Drive
San Antonio, TX 78231

Phone: 210-555-1234   **Fax:** 210-555-1235

Patient name: *Anthony Martin*   **Date:** *08/05/*

Address: *8674 Madien Way San Antonio, TX 78231*

Singular 2mg

#30

1 tab po qd

Refills: *1*

Dr.'s signature: *John Smith, MD*   **DEA #:** *AS123456*

Robert Kelly, MD
1234 Medical Drive
San Antonio, TX 78231

Phone: 210-555-1234   **Fax:** 210-555-1235

Patient name: _Kim Marie Williams_   **Date:** _08/05/_

Address: _9786 Bonjour Drive San Antonio, TX 78231_

Keflex 500mg

_#30_

1 cap po tid x 10 days

Refills: _0_

Dr.'s signature: _Robert Kelly, MD_   **DEA #:** _AS123456_

John Smith, MD
1234 Medical Drive
San Antonio, TX 78231

Phone: 210-555-1234   **Fax:** 210-555-1235

Patient name: _Jocelyn Adams_   **Date:** _08/05/_

Address: _4532 Santiago Boulevard San Antonio, TX 78231_

Z-pak

#1 pak

2 tabs po today then 1 tab qd x 4 days

Refills: _0_

Dr.'s signature: _John Smith, MD_   **DEA #:** _AS123456_

John Smith, MD
1234 Medical Drive
San Antonio, TX 78231

Phone: 210-555-1234   **Fax:** 210-555-1235

Patient name: _Julie Conover_   **Date:** _08/05/_

Address: _456723 Purple Lane San Antonio, TX 78231_

Bactroban Cream

#1 tube

Apply to affected area bid ud

Refills: _0_

Dr.'s signature: _John Smith, MD_   **DEA #:** _AS123456_

Herbert Lewis, MD
1234 Medical Drive
San Antonio, TX 78231

Phone: 210-555-1234   **Fax:** 210-555-1235

Patient name: _Carolann Contreras_   **Date:** _08/05/_

Address: _7701 Flaca Avenue San Antonio, TX 78231_

Glyburide 5mg

#30

1 tab po qd

Refills: _0_

Dr.'s signature: _Herbert Lewis, MD_   **DEA #:** _AS123456_

John Smith, MD
1234 Medical Drive
San Antonio, TX 78231

Phone: 210-555-1234   **Fax:** 210-555-1235

Patient name: _Christopher Cousin_   **Date:** _08/05/_

Address: _San Antonio, TX 78231_

Glucophage 500mg

#30

1 tab bid po qd

Refills: _3_

Dr.'s signature: _John Smith, MD_   **DEA #:** _AS123456_

John Smith, MD
1234 Medical Drive
San Antonio, TX 78231

Phone: 210-555-1234 **Fax:** 210-555-1235

Patient name: _Sylvia Ramirez_ **Date:** _08/05/_

Address: _2143 Sunnyside Drive San Antonio, TX 78231_

Valtrex 500mg

_#30_

1 tab po qd

Refills: _3_

Dr.'s signature: _John Smith, MD_ **DEA #:** _AS123456_

John Smith, MD
1234 Medical Drive
San Antonio, TX 78231

Phone: 210-555-1234   **Fax:** 210-555-1235

Patient name: _Kathryn Barnes_   **Date:** _08/05/_

Address: _81 Loop Rise San Antonio, TX 78231_

Atarax 25mg

#30

1 tab po q6 hours prn allergies

Refills: _1_

Dr.'s signature: _John Smith, MD_   **DEA #:** _AS123456_

Herbert Lewis, MD
1234 Medical Drive
San Antonio, TX 78231

Phone: 210-555-1234 **Fax:** 210-555-1235

Patient name: _Christina Prosser_ **Date:** _08/05/_

Address: _8764 Foxy Lane San Antonio, TX 78231_

Humulin N

#2 boxes

Inject 15 units sq tid ac

Refills: _0_

Dr.'s signature: _Herbert Lewis, MD_ **DEA #:** _AS123456_

Be sure to cut out the windows
so you can see the numbers!

F o l d   H e r e

To convert

Multiply by

To:

| 30 ml |

From:

Divide by

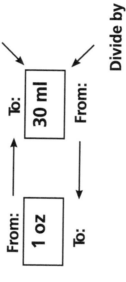

From:

| 1 oz |

To:

To use the converter, slide the inner card
up and down until you find the conversion factor you need.
If you are converting from the unit of measure
on the left to the unit of measure on the right,
multiply by the number in the box on the right.
If you are converting from the unit of measure
on the right to the unit of measure on the left,
divide by the number in the box on the right

Ex: 3.25 oz = _____ ml

Slide the inner card until you find the conversion factor
you need. To convert from oz to ml
multiply by the number in the right hand box, 30.

$3.25 \times 30 = 97.5$

The answer is 97.5ml

Ex: 375 ml = _____ oz

To convert from ml to oz, divide by the number
in the right hand box, 30.

375 divided by 30 = 12.5

The answer is 12.5 oz

F o l d   H e r e

T a p e   H e r e

Fold Here

1 L	1000 ml
1 ml	1 cc
1 ml	15 gtt
1 oz	30 ml
1 pt	473 ml
1 qt	946 ml
1 pt	16 oz
1 qt	32oz

Fold Here

1 kg	1000 g
1 g	1000 mg
1 mg	1000 mcg
1 lb	454 gm
1 kg	2.2 lbs
1 oz	30 gm
1 gr	60mg/65mg
1 lb	16 oz